Culturally Sensitive Oral Healthcare

Quintessentials of Dental Practice – 35
General Dentistry – 1

Culturally Sensitive Oral Healthcare

By
Crispian Scully CBE
Nairn H F Wilson CBE

Editor-in-Chief: Nairn H F Wilson
Editor General Dentistry: Nairn H F Wilson

Quintessence Publishing Co. Ltd.
London, Berlin, Chicago, Paris, Milan, Barcelona, Istanbul,
São Paulo, Tokyo, New Delhi, Moscow, Prague, Warsaw

British Library Cataloguing-in Publication Data

Scully, Crispian
  Culturally sensitive oral healthcare. - (Quintessentials of dental of dental practice; 35.
  Clinical practice; 1)
  1. Dentistry - Social aspects - Great Britian 2. Dentistry - Religious aspect
  3. Minorities - Dental care - Great Britian
  I. Title II. Wilson, Nairn H.F.
  617.6´0089´00941

ISBN 1850971188

ISBN 1-85097-118-8

Foreword

A striking feature of health in contemporary Britain is the diversity among different ethnic groups. Cultural differences may be important in risk of disease. They are also important in contacts with the healthcare system: no less for oral disease than for other health problems. An understanding of the culture of patients, and of differences between healthcare provider and recipient, is vital for quality healthcare that meets people's needs. This book is, therefore, timely and necessary and much to be welcomed.

Professor Sir Michael Marmot KBE
MBBS, MPH, PhD, FRCP, FFPHM
Director, International Centre for Health and Society
Professor of Epidemiology and Public Health, University College London
Chairman, Commission on Social Determinants of Health

Preface

Dentists and dental care professionals (DCPs) may work in countries foreign to them, or provide care to refugees or other patients who have immigrated into their country of work. History shows centuries of conflict and the movement of populations in many, if not most parts of the world. Colonisation and subsequent decolonisation, wars, natural disasters, competition for limited resources and the natural desire of human beings to explore new worlds, have resulted in enormous changes, especially in recent times. There is scarcely a country that has been exempt from such changes and, even in the 21st century, conflicts and disasters seem set to continue, with the likelihood of further population shifts and more immigration into countries that provide a safe haven. The world is also shrinking, with globalisation following tremendous technological advances, facilitating travel and communication. Most countries, in particular the so-called developed countries, are thus becoming increasingly culturally, ethnically and racially diverse. This trend is certain to continue and probably to escalate. The many diverse people of the world are thus now widely distributed, living in either fully integrated or multicultural societies. Similarly, people travel widely, with increasing exposure to other cultures.

Modern healthcare delivery demands that the religious, cultural and ethical beliefs of patients be considered as a part of their treatment. There is therefore an increasing need to understand other cultures. Culture is a term used to refer to shared patterns, meanings and behaviours of a social group. Understanding and respecting differing cultures, religions, ethnicities and values within society is increasingly recognised as critical to good quality healthcare provision. All healthcare providers (HCPs), including dentists and dental care professionals (DCPs), increasingly need to understand the culture of their patient. Some HCPs have been tardy in appreciating the importance and the improved quality of care that comes from patient-centred care. Each dental patient is an individual with personal views about their illness. These views may not concur with those of the HCP. Patients have personal wishes, needs and concerns that demand the understanding and respect of the HCP. Patients increasingly and rightly expect to be offered choice, not just about when and where they receive treatment, but also about what kind of treatment they receive, how it will be delivered and by whom. Extending choice is especially important in responding to the needs and preferences of an increasingly diverse population. Also, it is increasingly recognised that involving patients as full partners in decisions about treatment leads to better health outcomes. Many studies have shown that patients' attitudes to the benefits and risks of treatment, and the extent to which they find adverse effects tolerable, can differ markedly from assumptions made by HCPs. Patients' beliefs and views are key influences as to whether and how they accept treatment. Patients are generally much more likely to complete treatment if their views and preferences have been recognised and taken into account, and they have been active partners in decisions. Client-centred, contemporary dental practice will be realised only if clinicians are equipped to interact with and provide care for clients of varied cultures and cultural backgrounds.

We work in a multicultural society. For example, in 2006 in London, about 300 languages were spoken, and more than one in three of the population was from minority ethnic populations. There are now more new registered dentists in the UK who have qualified overseas than there are those who have qualified in the UK and, furthermore, many of the latter are not of Anglo-Saxon British culture. Few places in the world are as religiously, ethnically and culturally diverse as the UK. Experience in London and other centres, reinforced by teaching and working with colleagues from a multitude of backgrounds, has made us particularly aware of the need for formal guidance for dentists and dental care professionals (DCPs). This need extends to dentists and DCPs from many different cultures. Despite this, there still appears to be a need for more formal information for dentists and DCPs.

We have attempted to address this need by developing this book to provide members of the dental team with a reference source to culturally sensitive care in everyday clinical practice. This is not a text about technical dentistry. Neither is this book intended to cover the orofacial problems that can affect people of various cultures and lifestyles, although they are mentioned where relevant. This book is about patient care.

The knowledge base to be culturally sensitive is enormous. Lists of cultural traits and religious customs and beliefs can help, but inevitably give a very false impression of uniformity. Thus, in making reference to such lists, it is crucial to remember that there is considerable variation within every cultural and religious group and to avoid stereotyping. The information given applies only to certain patients. It is not a recipe for all solutions: we simply provide guidelines as a starting point for individualising dental healthcare.

Individuals' views, practices, needs and wishes vary widely and can be influenced by religion, ethnicity, educational, socioeconomic, acculturational and other factors.

This book is presented in three sections. The first section covers the many aspects of culturally sensitive healthcare, the second section outlines features of various religions and faiths and the third discusses cultural groups. In the second and third sections, topics have been arranged alphabetically for convenience. We do not attempt to be comprehensive. Cross-referencing has been essential.

We have been strongly influenced by the excellent works of Michael Marmot, Alix Henley and Judith Schott, and by Raman Bedi, and must pay tribute to their ideals and efforts. We have also sought advice from advisors who have been listed. We are grateful to all for their comments. We are particularly grateful to Arun Haricharan, who works in the community providing oral healthcare to a wide range of peoples, for his generous reading and criticism of the text. We are also grateful to John Huw Evans for his diligence in checking the various websites for the latest URLs (accessed October 2005). We, however remain responsible for any errors. Indeed, we are acutely aware that, despite our efforts to the contrary, what we have written could be regarded by some as incorrect, or unnecessarily or incorrectly generalising or stereotyping. We have tried throughout to emphasise the enormous diversity in cultures, health beliefs and practices. Individuals may subscribe to all, some or none of these. The only way to provide culturally sensitive healthcare is to listen and be sensitive to each and every patient and, when appropriate, ask about personal needs and wishes.

Individual interpretations of religions and the influence of cultural practices means there are no universal healthcare practices and beliefs in any religion or culture. Assumptions are no alternative to seeking and respecting the wishes of individual patients.

Although we are based in the United Kingdom, we hope that our efforts will help improve culturally sensitive oral healthcare worldwide.

Crispian Scully
Nairn Wilson
London, 2006

Advisors

Advisor	Affiliation	Topics
Oslei paes de Almeida	University of Campinas, Brazil	Latin Americans
Tereza Belai	Eastman Dental Institute London, UK	Eritreans Ethiopeans
Toshio Deguchi	Matsumoto Dental University Japan	Japanese
Andrew Eder	Eastman Dental Institute London, UK	Judaism
Mohammed El-Maaytah	Eastman Dental Institute London, UK	Arabs Islam
Channa Jayasena	The Hammersmith Hospital London, UK	Jainism Indians
Navdeep Kumar	Eastman Dental Institute London, UK	Indians Sikhism
Rachel Leeson	Eastman Dental Institute London, UK	Christianity
Serdar Mutlu	Istanbul University, Turkey	Kurds Turks
Yuan-ling (Paula) Ng	Eastman Dental Institute London, UK	Buddhism Chinese Confucianism Taoism
Mohammed Maryoud	Eastman Dental Institute London, UK	Islam Somalis
Naresh Pindolia	Eastman Dental Institute London, UK	Hinduism Indians Jainism
Cynthia Pine	University of Liverpool, UK	Caribbeans
Rene Ponciano	Eastman Dental Institute London, UK	Filipinos
Keith Shear	University of Birmingham, UK	Africans African religions

Mervyn Shear	University of the Western Cape	Africans
	South Africa	African religions
Prasanna Sooriakumaran	Royal Surrey County Hospital	Hinduism
	Guildford, UK	Indians
David Wiesenfeld	Royal Melbourne Hospital	Australasians
	Australia	

Acknowledgement

We are grateful to Taylor & Francis Publishers (London) and to Drs Scully, Flint, Porter and Moos, for permission to reproduce some illustrations from their Atlas of Oral and Maxillofacial Diseases (2004).

Contents

Section 1
Diversity, Cultural Considerations and Definitions

Aim

The aim of this section is to offer an overview of aspects of culturally sensitive healthcare, with an emphasis on culturally sensitive oral healthcare provision.

Outcome

Having read this section, readers should be more aware of the immediate steps needed to make their patient management more culturally sensitive, before exploring the religious, cultural and other aspects of healthcare dealt with in more depth in subsequent sections.

Introduction

Many areas of the world are short of resources, and this applies especially to the tropics, and areas fraught by natural and man-made disasters. Difficult environments, inadequate nutrition and insufficient healthcare are common in resource-poor areas, leading to enumerable health and other problems. The fact that there are disparities in health between different ethnic, cultural or other groups is not new.

Cultures and Cultural Considerations

Culture (Latin colere; to inhabit, to cultivate, or to honour) is a term that refers to patterns of human activity and the symbolic structures that give such activity significance. Culture can be seen as consisting of three elements:

- Values – comprise ideas about what seems important and guides the rest of the culture.
- Norms – consist of expectations of how people should behave in different situations. Each culture has different methods, sanctions, of enforcing its norms, which vary with their importance. Norms that a society enforces formally have the status of laws.
- Artifacts – things, or material culture, which derive from the culture's values and norms.

1

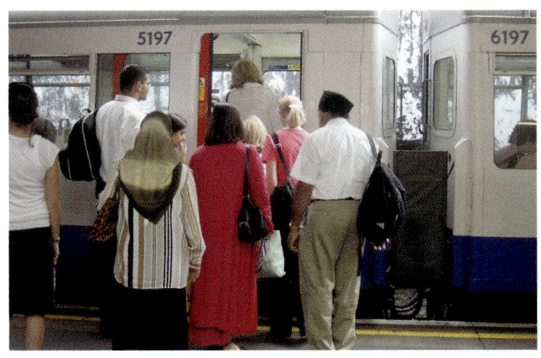

Fig 1-1 London: a multi-cultural society.

Cultures can differ in a number of ways. Cultural differences are based on combinations of values, norms and artifacts. This has many implications for healthcare.

Cultures are often based on some sort of religion or faith, or similar basis developed for inculcating and preserving established or 'correct' cultural behaviour. Groups of immigrants, exiles or minorities often form cultural associations or clubs to preserve their own cultural roots in the face of a surrounding (generally more locally-dominant) culture. On a broader scale, many countries market their cultural heritage internationally, both in the promotion of tourism and in cultural development abroad.

Cultural changes can and do occur – in particular in response to the environment (including education and socioeconomic status), to inventions (and other internal influences), and to contact with other cultures. When this affects an individual or groups of people, it is often termed 'acculturation'.

Multicultural societies are now common in many parts of the world, with increasing numbers of immigrants and their families seeking local access to culturally sensitive routine oral healthcare provision (Fig 1-1).

In addition, the healthcare professions have become much more multicultural, given increasing numbers graduates from different cultures and backgrounds, with many being more aware of religious and cultural issues than some older members of the professions. It is clear that healthcare professionals in a multicultural society must function across cultural divides.

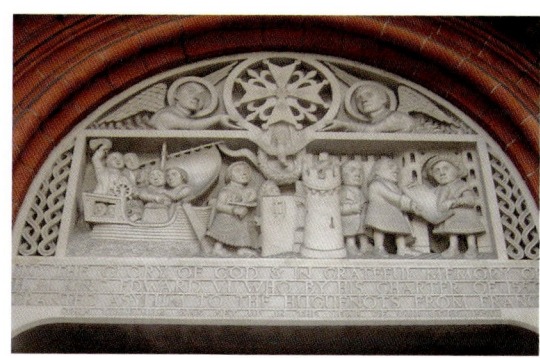

Fig 1-2 Plaque commemorating migration to the UK in part centuries.

The health manifestations of culture are significant and determine patient behaviours. Immigration is not a new phenomenon and is unlikely to cease. Migrants from diverse social, economic and educational backgrounds arrive in other countries for a variety of reasons. Many are refugees fleeing war, political upheaval, persecution, natural disasters or deprivation in their home countries. Some are joining families from which they have been separated for years. Yet others come seeking education or financial advantage, or to provide or seek work. Evidence suggests that the desire or need to emigrate from various places around the world is unlikely to diminish (Fig 1-2).

Many immigrants arrive with inadequate economical support and language skills and tend to suffer social exclusion and inequality of healthcare provision. In many countries there is inequality of healthcare provision to a minority of the population who are the most deprived and socially excluded: this minority is often related to ethnic or cultural differences.

Cultural considerations in oral healthcare are increasingly important. As in healthcare in general, dentists and dental care professionals (DCPs) are increasingly expected to be familiar with ethnic, cultural and religious issues that impact on healthcare provision, and to be willing and able to treat patients belonging to different religious and ethnic groups in ways that will not cause embarrassment, let alone distress through breaches of religious and ethnic groups' taboos. Dentists and DCPs may work in countries foreign to them, or provide care to patients who have immigrated into their country of work. In either case, it is important for the dentist and DCP to understand and recognise the culture of patients. Most members of the dental team work in

3

their home countries and will have experienced interactions with new immigrants, those who have acculturated, and individuals who are descendants of people who may have immigrated some time ago.

In many societies, it is suggested that the need for culturally sensitive oral healthcare provision has traditionally tended to be relatively limited or ignored, with relatively small numbers of patients in religious and ethnic minority groups having tended to seek dental and related oral healthcare from HCPs within their group. This may have involved a number of barriers such as cost, fear, mistrust, the need to travel long distances at inconvenient times, or the absence of dental HCPs able and willing to accommodate specific cultural and ethnic needs. The exception is hospital-based and salaried dental services, which individuals of all religious and ethnic groups tend to access for emergency and possibly specialist care. Culturally sensitive healthcare is a phrase used to describe a healthcare system that, in addition to being accessible, respects the beliefs, attitudes and cultural lifestyles both of the patient and, as a consequence, is sensitive to issues including culture, race, gender, sexual orientation, social class and economic situation. At the most simple level, it is easy to offend by asking for a 'Christian' name (from someone who may not be Christian) rather than a 'personal' ('first') name.

Cultural competency is the understanding that we all have different values that affect the way we view our health and healthcare, and how we view the world. It implies the ability to successfully navigate through other cultures while understanding, appreciating, making comparisons to, and moving beyond stereotypes, while remaining sensitive to one's own cultural elements and those of other persons. The goal is to provide the best care possible to each individual patient. Culturally competent care requires more than simply a knowledge of other cultures; it involves attitudes and skills as well.

Once attuned to the cultural beliefs of the patient, the healthcare professional can become a more effective HCP, and a more positive health advocate. Thus healthcare is offered in a way that respects and recognises different religions and cultural needs.

Families
In Anglo-American cultures there is a high proportion of nuclear families and, increasingly, lone-parent families and families in which parents live together but are not married, including some single-sex families. Independence is a characteristic of these cultures.

The family structure is a significant feature of cultures where the extended family is more common than the nuclear family. In extended families, the elders act as role models, are in control, and are respected. Often the family decides where to seek healthcare, whether this be from a HCP, a traditional healer, or even a neighbour. They also may decide whether to comply with appointments and accept medication and other treatments.

The perceived advantages and disadvantages of different family systems are highlighted in Table 1-1.

It is important to be aware of the various possibilities in a specific culture. But it is equally important to recognise that individuals within a culture may not conform to the cultural norms, in particular if living in a different country or community and if they have undergone acculturation.

Table 1-1 **Some perceived advantages and disadvantages of extended and nuclear families**

Perceptions	Extended families	Nuclear families
Features	Strong family, higher social control, lower individualism.	Weak family, lower social control, higher individualism.
Healthcare decision-making	Often by older male, more educated family member, or more wealthy family member.	Often by individual. Parent, spouse or partner may be consulted by the individual.
Advantages	Limited involvement in aberrant behaviour. Strong family support. Infrequent loneliness.	Less conformation. More freedom.
Disadvantages	Less freedom. More conformation.	Tendency to aberrant behaviour. Less family support. Frequent loneliness.

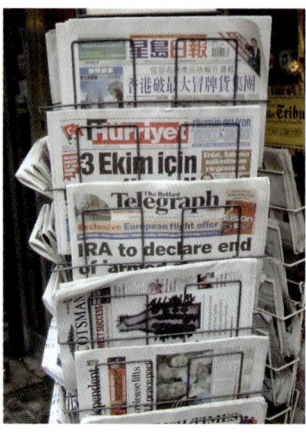

Fig 1-3 Diversity in the UK as demonstrated visibly by newspapers in different languages.

Diversity

Populations are diverse, and are becoming increasingly more diverse in many, if not most, countries. Section 3 of this book gives a broad outline of the various cultural groups of the world, highlighting diversity in and between most countries, in particular the developed countries of the world. Diversity extends beyond the colour of a person's skin and religion to age, socio-economic status, sexual orientation, gender identification and lifestyle differences. Thus, there is both visible and invisible diversity (Fig 1-3). Furthermore, diversity may decrease or even increase in immigrant populations as they acculturate in the dominant culture of their host country (Fig 1-4).

Cultural, religious and healthcare views can be diverse and can also be difficult to interpret and can change. Frequently, the level of devotion and adherence to a cultural or religious practice will vary between patients and over time, depending on factors such as age, events and circumstances. The view of a specific cultural or religious group may also differ, depending on the denomination or sect, the leader in a particular area and other powerful influences, including education and socio-economic status.

In view of the enormous diversity in cultures, religions and faiths, and health beliefs and practices, it is not possible to discuss these here from the traditional perspective as seen in the home country. Individuals may subscribe to all, some or none. The only way to provide culturally sensitive healthcare is to be aware, listen and be sensitive to each and every patient and, when appropriate, ask about personal needs and wishes. Assumptions are no alternative to seeking and respecting the wishes of individual patients.

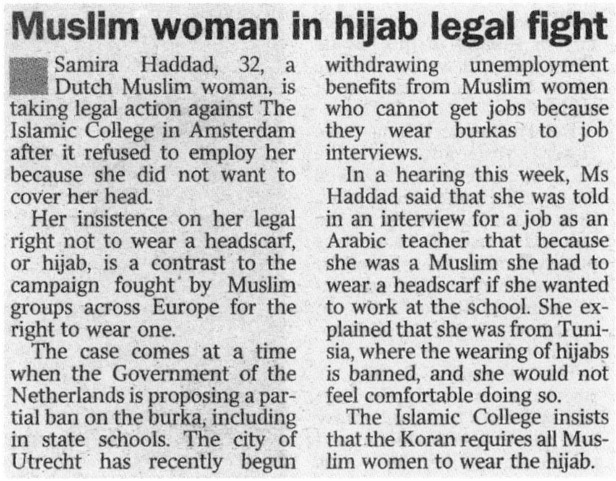

Muslim woman in hijab legal fight

Samira Haddad, 32, a Dutch Muslim woman, is taking legal action against The Islamic College in Amsterdam after it refused to employ her because she did not want to cover her head.

Her insistence on her legal right not to wear a headscarf, or hijab, is a contrast to the campaign fought by Muslim groups across Europe for the right to wear one.

The case comes at a time when the Government of the Netherlands is proposing a partial ban on the burka, including in state schools. The city of Utrecht has recently begun withdrawing unemployment benefits from Muslim women who cannot get jobs because they wear burkas to job interviews.

In a hearing this week, Ms Haddad said that she was told in an interview for a job as an Arabic teacher that because she was a Muslim she had to wear a headscarf if she wanted to work at the school. She explained that she was from Tunisia, where the wearing of hijabs is banned, and she would not feel comfortable doing so.

The Islamic College insists that the Koran requires all Muslim women to wear the hijab.

Fig 1-4 Newspaper article showing diversity and conformity in Europe.

Definitions

The debate on terminology pertinent to diversity and equality is constantly evolving. Some of the more common terms are noted above, but others include the following:

- *'Acculturation'* is the process whereby a minority group, as a result of exposure to a different system, modifies its social norms, attitudes, values and behaviours, variously relinquishing or retaining some of its original characteristics.
- *'Affirmative action'* refers to a set of public policies and initiatives designed to eliminate past and present discrimination based on race, colour, religion, sex, or national origin, and thereby to provide equal opportunity to individuals and groups of individuals that have been systematically discriminated against.
- *'Asylum seeker'* is a person who has applied for refugee status and who is awaiting a decision on residency.
- *'Culture'* refers to shared patterns, meanings and behaviours of a social group. It generally refers to patterns of human activity and the symbolic structures that give such activity significance.
- *'Cultural competency'* implies ability to navigate through other cultures while understanding, appreciating, making comparisons to, moving beyond stereotypes, and remaining sensitive to one's own cultural elements and those of other people.
- *'Cultural relativism'* is defined as the view that all ethical truth is relative to a specified culture.
- *'Culturally sensitive healthcare'* is a phrase used to describe a healthcare system that is accessible and respects the beliefs, attitudes and cultural lifestyles

7

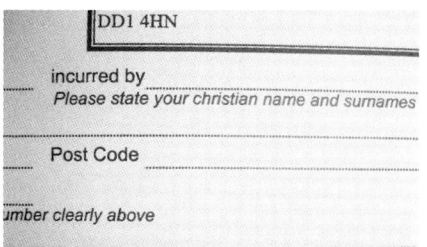

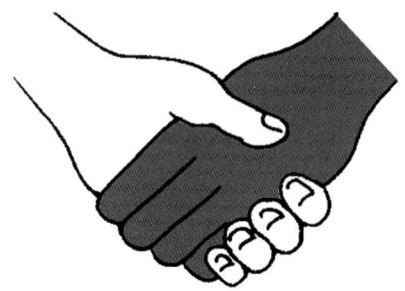

Fig 1-5 A National Health Services form showing insensitivity over requests for the personal name.

Fig 1-6 Race is not simply related to skin colour.

both of the professional and the patient, and is sensitive, amongst other things, to issues related to culture, race, gender, sexual orientation, social class and economic situation.

- *'Diversity'* may involve differences in ethnicity, and differences in social factors such as regional, age, religious, urban/rural or social class differences.

- *'Ethnicity'* is a description for a number of attributes such as genetic inheritance and ancestry, religion and culture (including diet, language, dress and lifestyle). 'Ethnicity' is defined in the UK as 'a group with a long-shared history and a distinct culture' (1983: Mandla v Lee. House of Lords).

- *'Ethnocentrism'* is the tendency to judge the customs of other societies by the standards of one's own ethnographic present.

- *'Eurocentrism'* is the practice of consciously (or unconsciously) privileging the culture of Europe over other cultures (Fig 1-5).

- *'Generalisation'* is the assumption about a group that leads to seeking further information about whether such assumption fits the individual.

- *'Institutional racism or structural racial discrimination'* is racial discrimination by governments, corporations or other large organisations such as the police.

- *'Race'* equates with human biologic variation. Once simplistically related to colour of skin (caucasoid, negroid etc) (Fig 1-6), 'race' is now used as a definition of a population that looks different from the locally dominant (majority) culture and has a different ancestral root.

- *'Racial discrimination'* is giving or withholding privileges based on racial or ethnic stereotypes. 'Racial prejudice' is assuming that every individual's character can be adequately determined by racial or ethnic stereotypes.

- *'Racism'* is a form of persecution based on beliefs, practices, and institutions that negatively discriminate against people based solely on their perceived or ascribed race. The United Nations defines racism as 'any distinction, exclusion, restriction or preference based on race, colour, descent, or national or ethnic origin, which has the purpose or effect of nullifying or impairing the recognition, enjoyment or exercise, on an equal footing, of human rights and fundamental freedoms in the political, economic, social, cultural or any other field of public life'.
- *'Refugee'* is a person who has been granted refugee status.
- *'Religion'* is a belief in, worship of, or obedience to a supernatural power or powers considered to be divine or to have control of human destiny. Religion is often closely related to ethnicity.
- *'Reverse discrimination'* or reverse racism is the belief that measures designed to correct alleged racism, such as affirmative action, have in fact simply created new racist policies against the locally dominant groups.
- *'Stereotype'* is to categorise people based on an artificial construction of a certain group designed to impart the 'essence' of that group, which homogenises the group, ignoring and effacing individuality and difference (Fig 1-7).
- *'Vulnerable groups'* – Vulnerability and disadvantage are often caused by marginalisation in, and exclusion

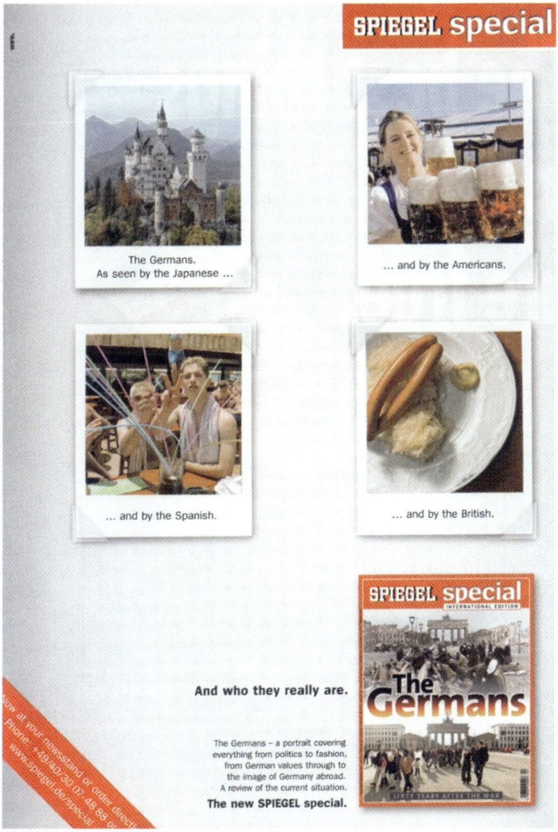

Fig 1-7 Stereotypes of one country and people as highlighted in the German magazine '*Der Spiegel*'.

9

from the socio-economic mainstream and decision-making processes and the lack of access, on an equal basis, to resources and opportunities.
- *'Xenophobia'*– dislike of foreign people.

Diseases Prevalent in New Immigrants from Resource-Poor Areas

In people living in, or immigrants newly arriving from, resource-poor areas, certain diseases may be especially prevalent. The approach to health provision in resource-poor areas is primarily curative rather than preventive.

In any population, disease can arise from the outcome of the interactions of three main factors:
- Genetics.
- Environment.
- Lifestyle.

Hereditary factors are especially important, as in sickle cell disease and glucose-6-phosphate dehydrogenase (G6PD) deficiency seen especially in persons of African or Asian origin, and thalassaemia, Behcet's disease and pemphigus seen particularly in persons from the Mediterranean littoral.

Environmental factors are most prevalent in resource-poor areas, in particular in war zones, where there have been natural disasters, in the developing world and in tropical regions. Thus poverty, malnutrition and bacterial infections such as tuberculosis (TB) and leprosy, viral infections such as hepatitis B, hepatitis C, and HIV, deep mycoses such as histoplasmosis, and parasitic diseases such as schistosomiasis, leishmaniasis and malaria may be cause for concern.

Lifestyle factors also predispose some groups to diseases. Many people in resource-poor areas have been traumatised, at least by relocation, if not by starvation and malnutrition, violence, natural disasters and bereavement. Stress and psychological trauma are common. Some disorders are related to poverty and lifestyle habits (e.g. infections, areca nut use and oral submucous fibrosis; tobacco chewing and oral cancer). Religious and cultural factors may also be at play - for example, veganism and subsequent vitamin B12 deficiency in Hindus.

Although resource-poor countries are managing to improve health and healthcare, diseases associated with unsanitary living conditions, minimal access to healthcare and inadequate diet continue to affect those in the lowest economic strata. Some of the health problems in immigrants may be modified during acculturation if there are changes in lifestyle and healthcare. Acculturation occurs to a variable extent and, sadly, may bring its own problems.

The Immigrant and Acculturation

Immigration can lead to a profound change in lifestyle and result in a range of behavioural changes in newcomers. Three main phases have been identified.

The First Phase

Since many diseases and other problems such as malnutrition are more prevalent in poverty- stricken areas, the 'acute phase' following immigration, in particular from the developing world, war zones and some tropical regions, attracts most concern. The serious and sometimes communicable nature of the illnesses with which new immigrants may present may be a potential public health threat. Other problems include violence in hostile communities and psychiatric reactions.

Generally speaking, new immigrants tend to:
• be of a different culture from the locally dominant community
• be young
• lack linguistic fluency
• be stressed and anxious
• be part of an extended family
• have low income
• have low standards of housing.

Social exclusion and barriers to healthcare are often present and can prevent access to care. Immigrants may also run into conflict with aspects of their new life, because of different views and values. In terms of health and healthcare, new immigrants may:
• lack understanding of healthcare system available to them
• lack awareness of preventive practices and screening
• have some reliance on traditional (folk) medicine
• have views on consent issues unaligned to local accepted thoughts and practice.

Cultural beliefs shape the perception and understanding of health and disease, and thus behaviours. Many immigrants come from healthcare systems that differ from western medicine, may not always be as advanced, and may

11

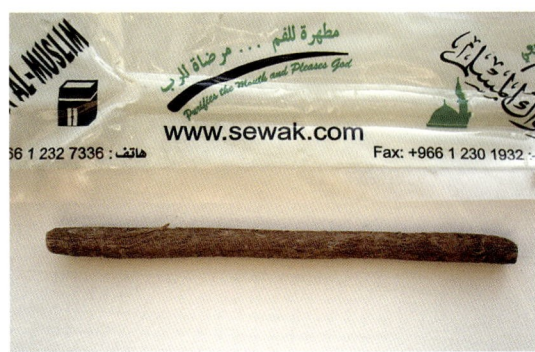

Fig 1-8 Miswak.

involve traditional remedies and healers. For example, some immigrant patients expect medication even for a minor illness, and are concerned if treatment does not include a prescription. Others routinely share prescriptions and over-the-counter (OTC) medications with friends and family.

Those coming from, in particular, countries in upheaval can suffer from a variety of health problems and post-traumatic stress syndrome. Some suffer from psychiatric disorders following persecution, racism or perceived racism. Depression and anxiety are common. Such factors, combined with the stigma associated with ill-health, possible social deprivation and the lack of family support networks, may prevent many from seeking healthcare. Amongst other problems, perinatal mortality rates may be high.

People coming from places where dentists have not been available, and branded oral healthcare products hardly affordable, may still practise traditional toothbrushing with, for example, miswaks (Fig 1-8) or salt. They may well lack understanding of the existence or roles of dental care services, let alone other healthcare resources.

A lack of understanding of the healthcare system can dissuade newcomers from attending to their health needs. Newcomers are confronted with understanding the complexity of healthcare in their new environment – decentralised structures, the principle of choice of healthcare providers, the need for health insurance, the emphasis on preventive health, and more. There can also be large differences in healthcare utilisation between different cultures, generating barriers to care. These may include:
• anxiety
• communication problems

- cultural beliefs
- denial
- cultural insensitivity on the part of HCPs
- lack of understanding
- work practices
- cost.

For the newcomer, this can result in:
- alienation
- mistrust.
- frustration
- wasted time
- poor treatment
- increased morbidity
- increased mortality.

Many newly arrived immigrants therefore suffer from lack of proper immunisations, let alone medical and dental healthcare. They often seek help only when emergency treatment is required.

The Second Phase
The second phase of immigration, transition, which typically occurs over at least five years, involves acculturation with modification of social norms, attitudes, values, behaviours and diet. Transition brings significant changes – not least in health behaviours and the use of healthcare services. The rate and degree of acculturation is largely influenced by:
- religion
- place of birth and degree of exposure to the majority culture
- age
- historic background
- socioeconomics
- education.

Most young immigrants become well integrated into the community to a far greater extent than their parents: this is most obvious in cultures in which religion does not vary significantly from that of the immigrants. Acculturation can also be influenced by the attitude of the majority culture. Uprooted, threatened cultures and religions may become increasingly conservative ('fundamental' or 'radical').

In transition, communicable diseases prevalent in the first stage of resettlement are generally brought under control. Conditions such as hypertension, diabetes and ischaemic heart disease may, however, become more prevalent through lifestyle factors such as lack of exercise, smoking and diet.

Psychological disorders, including conversion reactions, seizures and other post-traumatic stress sequelae tend to become more prevalent. The latter may arise from the stress of adjustment to a new culture, the burden of the past and separation from traditional family and cultural support systems, intergenerational conflict, and conflict with other cultures (sometimes originating from conflicts in the home country), domestic violence, gambling and substance abuse. Other problems that may arise with acculturation include the sequelae of changing names, which can lead to confusion and family strife.

Immigrants in transition tend to acquire skills in the language of the locally dominant culture, gain access to healthcare services and adapt increasingly to local health practices, yet may develop further problems.

The Third Phase

The third phase, 10 or more years after arrival, is typified by the resettled immigrant using the host country healthcare services, but suffering from a variety of chronic conditions linked, at least in part, to the consequences of resettlement and, in many cases, emotional difficulties arising from change or possibly break down in family structures. Lifestyle can also significantly influence disease. For example, in the United Kingdom, tobacco smoking is high in third-phase Bangladeshi men and in Caribbean men and women. Hypertension, coronary heart disease and diabetes are the most common consequences.

In some communities there can be heavy alcohol consumption with high rates of liver disease, cirrhoses and other concomitants. Similarly, the morbidity and mortality from cancers tend to be high. Drug abuse may be seen in some groups. Intergenerational conflicts can arise, with exclusion of older people and breakdown of family relationships and values. Occasionally, the consequences can be as dramatic as gang conflicts.

Immigrants in the third phase thus tend to have gained access to, and make use of, healthcare services, increasingly using the locally dominant culture language, and following westernised health practices. Concurrently, they acquire the lifestyles, habits and diseases of the culturally locally dominant community, often associated with breakdown of the extended family and

Table 1-2 **Diseases prevalent in black and minority ethnic (BME) people in developed countries in Europe**

Condition	Comment
Diabetes	Six times more common in South Asians and three times more common in Blacks than Whites
	High rates of non-insulin dependent diabetes mellitus in South Asian and Caribbean minorities
Cancers	Oral cancer rates high in South Asian, African groups and those of Celtic origin
Haemo-globinopathies	Sickle cell disease and trait prevalent in African,
	Caribbean and South Asian populations. Thalassaemia more common amongst people from Southern Europe, Middle East and South Asia
Mental illness	Common in all immigrant groups. Suicide rates high, especially in young women from South Asia
Tuberculosis	High incidence amongst peoples from South Asia, Eastern Europe and Africa. High mortality amongst people born in Ireland
Sexually transmitted infections (STIs)	HIV prevalent in immigrants from sub-Saharan Africa, and increasingly from India and Eastern Europe
Violence	BME people are prone to be victims of harassment, violence, and robbery. Black Caribbeans tend to be victims of serious crimes of violence in their communities

intergenerational conflicts. In contrast, some individuals and groups may choose to retain or even accentuate their ancestral heritage. In either case disparities in health and health beliefs may continue to exist between people of minority ethnic backgrounds and the culturally locally dominant population.

Disparities in Health and Determinants of Health

In many multicultural societies there are inequalities in health and in the determinants of health. Illustrative of these inequalities are the following findings from a recent study in London:

*   Non-White groups are more likely than White people to be living in poor quality housing. Black households are three times more likely to be classed as unfit homes compared to White households: this is especially a problem for Bangladeshis and Pakistanis. Bangladeshi and Black Caribbean elders are more likely to be living in social housing than White or Indian groups.
*   There are variations in school performance. Black Caribbean children perform less well than most other Black and Minority Ethnic (BME) children at school. Gypsy/Roma children and those of Travellers of Irish Heritage have the lowest attainment in schools. In contrast, Chinese and Indian children perform better than others in school
*   Non-White groups are twice as likely as White people to be unemployed.
*   Bangladeshis have four times the rate of unemployment (20%) compared to White British (5%). Black groups have the highest unemployment rates for the under 25-year-old age group, and Bangladeshi households also have the lowest gross hourly earnings and incomes.
*   There are variations in type of employment. Chinese and Indian people are as, or more likely, to be in professional and managerial positions as Whites. People in BME groups who have qualifications are far more likely to be in employment than are those without. Whites, Indians and Chinese people are more likely than other BME groups to have parents who are salaried.
*   There are significant health problems in, and barriers to healthcare for BME populations. BME populations are consistently less satisfied than Whites with healthcare services, in particular with primary care. NHS Direct and walk-in centers are underused by the BME population. One in six refugees has a health problem severe enough to affect their lives. Elders from BME populations are more likely than older Whites to report poor health. Many BME populations have a high prevalence of certain diseases compared to the culturally dominant population in, for example, Europe.

Oral Health in Minority Groups

Oral Health Beliefs

People of all cultures may have limited knowledge of the risk factors for common oral disease, including dental caries and periodontal disease. Such limitations in knowledge may extend to serious conditions including cancer, in particular, amongst those who have not had the luxury of effective education or a high level of socioeconomic support. This applies especially to immigrant groups who, in the early stages of acculturation, are unlikely to routinely visit a dentist or other HCP.

Furthermore, the perception of health and disease varies in different groups. For example, older Chinese subjects perceive themselves as being at low risk for periodontitis, but in reality have more objective signs of periodontitis than subjects of European descent of comparable age.

Oral Health Practices

In westernised cultures, regular oral hygiene using a toothbrush and toothpaste is the norm. The importance of oral hygiene is often appreciated by people who have had contact with Anglo-American cultures, but this is not always the case.

The miswak (meswak, siwak, muswaki, mefaka) is a stick made from the roots or twigs of various trees and is used commonly in Muslim countries in the Middle East, Asia, and Africa (Fig 1-8). The World Health Organization (WHO) has recommended and encouraged the use of these sticks as an effective and inexpensive tool for oral hygiene.

Miswaks are produced from Salvadora persica (Arak), Eucalyptus camaldulensis and other plants. Chemicals identified in Salvadora persica include:
• chlorides
• flavonoids
• fluoride
• salvadorine
• saponins
• silica
• sterols
• sulphur
• tannins
• trimethylamine
• vitamin C (ascorbic acid).

The plaque-removing properties of the miswak and conventional tooth-brush are similar. In some studies, the miswak has been superior. Miswak users, however, develop significantly more gingival recession and occlusal wear than do toothbrush users, and the teeth may develop a distinctive yel-low stain. Miswaks may have some anticaries activity by virtue of the fluo-ride content.

Azadirachta indica (Neem) is the basis of chewing sticks used in India and parts of Africa. Fagara zanthoxyloides is the basis of chewing sticks used in parts of West Africa; and, in the West Indies, 'chaw sticks' are made from the plant Gounia lupiloides.

Teeth are also cleaned in some cultures using tooth powders derived from a variety of sources, including charcoal, ash, silica and tobacco.

Tongue cleaning is another ancient habit used in some cultural groups such as Hindus and Chinese, while in others (including most westerners) it is a novel concept. It can help reduce oral malodour.

Oral and Dental Health
Present (urban or rural) and past (country of origin) geographic location can represent a significant oral health risk marker, with those from rural loca-tions in developing countries being most at risk.

Children from deprived backgrounds in most cultures, including some minor-ity ethnic groups, often display the most caries. Those with caries may be fur-ther disadvantaged by having higher levels of caries-associated microflora (*Strep-tococcus mutans* and lactobacilli), and a more frequent consumption of sugars.

Racial and socioeconomic status (SES) disparities in oral health are also strong determinants of tooth loss. For example, in the USA, African Americans and lower SES adults have relatively fewer remaining teeth and are more likely to receive a dental extraction once they enter the dental care system, given the same disease extent and severity, than are other groups.

Periodontal disease is more common in some socioeconomic and/or cul-tural groups, often because of inadequate oral hygiene, sometimes linked to smoking or smokeless tobacco use. Acute ulcerative gingivitis, typically an infection of adolescents and young adults, is seen particularly in debilitated malnourished children from resource-poor countries, in smokers, and in immunocompromised people.

Tobacco use is a risk factor for coronal and root caries, periodontal disease, gingival recession, and oral mucosal disease.

Lifestyle Habits Affecting Oral Health

A number of lifestyle habits, in addition to dietary variations, are implicated in disease pathogenesis, especially various chewing and smoking habits, in particular those involving tobacco.

Chewing products
• Areca nut
Areca chewing is a habit of around 20% of the world population, especially common in people from South and South East Asia. Following migration, the habit tends to remain prevalent amongst its practitioners. Common effects of betel use are brown or black tooth and mucosal staining, and possibly increased periodontal disease, but some protection against dental caries (Figs 1-9 to 1-11). Submucous fibrosis (oral submucous fibrosis: OSMF) is also related to the use of areca nuts found in Pan masala and Gutkha. It is predominantly a disease of adults from the Indian sub-continent. Tight ver-

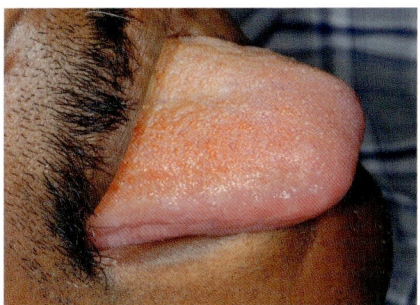

Fig 1-9 Betel staining of the tongue.

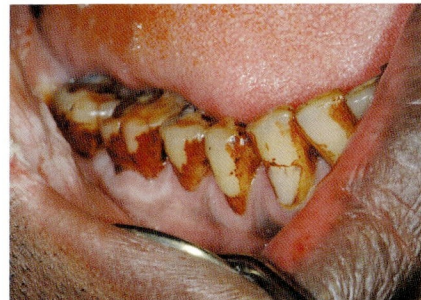

Fig 1-10 Betel staining of the teeth.

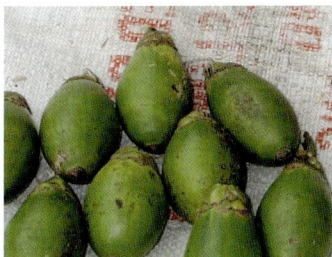

Fig 1-11 Betel nuts.

19

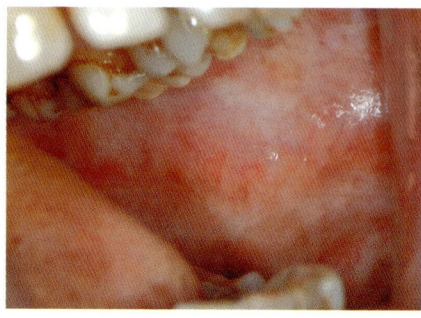

Fig 1-12 Oral submucous fibrosis.

tical bands in the buccal mucosa may progress to severely restricted oral opening (Fig 1-12). OSMF can also affect the palate or tongue. There is a malignant potential – carcinoma develops possibly in up to 8%. The carcinogenic effects of the betel quid, as are discussed below, appear related mainly to the tobacco content.

• Coca
Coca leaf chewing, seen in South America and in Java, India and Sri Lanka, involves the use of leaves from the shrub Erythroxylum coca, which release the stimulant alkaloid cocaine. Abuse of cocaine is seen in several cultures and may occasionally cause mucosal burns.

• Cola
Cola (kola) nut chewing is seen especially in people from West and Central Africa. The cola nut, from Cola acuminate, Cola verticillara or Cola nitida trees, releases stimulant alkaloids such as caffeine and theobromine. Oral complications have not been reported, but cola-containing beverages may cause dental erosion.

• Gums
Gums from the latex of several plants are customarily chewed in various cultures and, if sugar-free, can reduce dental caries.

• Khat
Chewing khat (qat) from the leaves of a cultivated, alkaloid shrub (Catha edulis), a habit mainly seen in peoples from the Arabian Peninsula and eastern Africa, is a stimulant due to the alkaloids, tannins, cathinone, cathine and norephedrine released. Oral effects include a low caries rate, an inverse relationship between periodontal pocket depths and the chewing side, tem-

poromandibular joint dysfunction, keratosis of the buccal mucosa, and occasional cancers. Shammah may have similar effects.

• Tobacco
Tobacco, whether chewed (smokeless tobacco) or smoked in various forms is implicated in many diseases – both systemic and oral, and often of a serious nature such as malignant neoplasms. It is the habit most associated with ill health. There are high levels of tobacco smoking in some ethnic groups.

Tobacco-associated problems include tooth stains, malodour, acute necrotising ulcerative gingivitis and other periodontal conditions, smoker's melanosis, burns and keratotic patches, black hairy tongue, nicotinic stomatitis, palatal erosions, leukoplakia, epithelial dysplasia and squamous-cell carcinoma, impaired healing after exodontia, surgery and periodontal treatment and implant failure.

Lifestyle Habits Implicated in Cancer
Tobacco use and excess alcohol consumption are the major risk factors for cancers of the oral cavity and pharynx. Marijuana (cannabis) use may also play a role in some oral cancers, though sometimes it is mixed with tobacco. The risks from tobacco and alcohol are synergistic, and heavy smokers (40 or more cigarettes/day) and heavy drinkers (30 or more drinks per week) have nearly 40 times the risk of developing oral cancer than abstainers.

Tobacco
Leukoplakia-like lesions and oral cancer may be induced by all forms of tobacco. Cross-sectional studies show a higher prevalence rate of leukoplakia, a potentially malignant disease, among smokers, with a dose-response relationship between tobacco use and oral leukoplakia, and intervention studies show a regression of the lesion after stopping the smoking habit. The overall risk of oral cancer among smokers is seven to 10 times higher than for those who never smoked. In a large-scale 10-year longitudinal survey in India, involving annual examination of 12,217 individuals, all new cancers that arose during follow-up were among tobacco users.

Smoking of bidi(s) made of hand-rolled tobacco wrapped in tendu leaf is a known risk factor for oral and pharyngeal cancer, common in Indians, and is also associated with a significantly higher mortality compared with tobacco chewing. Reverse smoking (holding the burning end of cigarettes or cigars within the oral cavity) is seen in parts of India and South America and in the Philippines, and is strongly associated with palatal lesions that carry a high risk of progressing to cancer. Age-adjusted mortality among reverse chutta (coarsely prepared cheroot) smokers is twice that of non-smokers. Smokeless tobacco (ST) use is common in Asia, and increasingly in the West. Traditional forms of ST use include betel quid, tobacco with lime and tobacco tooth powder. Pregnant women who use ST have a threefold increased risk of stillbirth and a two- to threefold increased risk of having a low birthweight infant.

Quid or paan (pan) is a mixture of substances placed in the mouth or actively chewed over an extended period. The specific components of this product vary between communities and individuals, but it usually contains tobacco and/or areca nut. Slaked lime may be added, and all is wrapped in a betel leaf. Addition of ST to the areca quid raises the relative oral cancer risk of the product by nearly 15 times.

Other ST products which carry significant mutagenicity are toombak (used in the Sudan), shammah (used in Saudi Arabia and North Africa), powdered tobacco and alkali mixtures such as nass/naswar (used in northern and central Asia and in Pakistan), khaini – a mixture of ST and lime (used in Nepal and Bihar state of India) – and boiled/sweetened ST called zarda (mostly used by people from Bangladesh). Maras powder is a kind of smokeless tobacco prepared from a mixture of ash and the powder obtained from the leaves of a tobacco plant in Turkey.

In the West, ST is also available – as oral snuff or in moist pouches. 'Snuff dipper's cancer' is especially prevalent in the Southern states of the USA and, despite the controversy as to the carcinogenicity of Swedish snuff ('snus'), retrospective studies have shown that users are indeed at high risk of cancer at the site of placement.

Alcohol
Increased alcohol consumption is associated with a risk of oral cancer and, for many countries follows a similar pattern to tobacco use. In 'alcohol-related' cancers, this is most seen in men in France, Italy and New Zealand. The differences in oral cancer incidence in African Americans have been attributed largely to heavy alcohol consumption, particularly amongst smokers.

Diets rich in fresh fruits and vegetables and vitamin A have a protective effect on oral cancer and precancer.

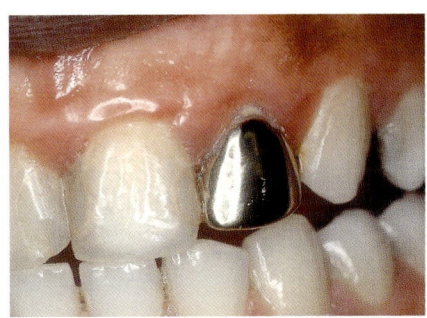

Fig 1-13 A gold crown placed as tooth jewellery.

Ethnic differences in cancer and cancer care
There is marked inter-country variation in both the incidence and mortality from oral cancer. In addition, there is also evidence of intracountry ethnic differences that have been attributed mainly to specific risk factors such as tobacco (smoking and smokeless) and alcohol. In the British Isles, for example, there are high levels of smoking and tobacco chewing in some minority ethnic groups, and also high levels of tobacco and alcohol use in some areas with high rates of oral cancer, such as Scotland and Ireland. However, dietary and genetic factors may also play a part.

Traditional Practices Affecting Oral Health
Traditional practices that persist today in various cultures include deliberate mutilation of hard or soft tissues.

Hard-tissue mutilation
Tooth mutilation and evulsion has been reported from several parts of the world, especially the developing world, in particular Africa. In the West, dentists are not infrequently approached to place gold crowns or restorations for aesthetic reasons alone – tooth jewellery (Fig 1-13). A number of cultures deliberately chip or reshape teeth. In parts of Uganda, Tanzania and Nigeria the operation of ebino, or 'false teeth', refers to the extraction of deciduous canine tooth buds when gingival swellings appear during the eruption of the primary canine teeth in infants. A similar practice in Somalia is 'Ilko dacowo'.

Tooth staining is another practice in some indigenous peoples in Peru and Ecuador, Vietnam, Laos, Thailand, Indonesia, the Philippines and Africa. In Nigeria for example, some people stain their teeth with flowers of Solanum incanum or Nicotania tabacum.

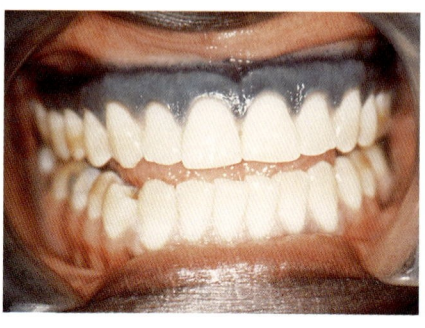

Fig 1-14 Gingival tattoo.

Soft-tissue mutilation
Facial and oral piercing is common in westernised societies, but also seen elsewhere, mainly in Africa and South America. Temporary mutilation by piercing is seen in Hindus as part of the religious ceremony Thapasyam.

Facial scarring is seen in many tribes in tropical Africa. Tattoos are also not uncommonly seen in some cultures. Tattoos on the face or elsewhere on the head and neck are seen in Maori, Nigeria and Cameroon, some Bedouins, and in some western cultures. Lip tattooing is seen mainly in North Africa. In Nigeria some people have the lip or gingivae tattooed before marriage, usually without local anaesthesia, using thorns of Balanites aegyptiaca and a mixture of charcoal and seeds of Acacia nilotica var. tomentosa as pigments. Maxillary blue-black gingival tattooing is seen in some female Muslims in North Africa and the Middle East (Fig 1-14). In some East African groups, children have uvulectomy in the belief that their health will be improved.

More detail on traditional practices is available elsewhere (see Wilson et al., 1992).

Traditional Healing
Traditional healers are commonplace in some cultures, especially in the developing world and associated with certain religions, in particular those of African or Chinese background. The concept of HCPs may be quite alien to such peoples. Alternatively, HCPs may complement the administrations of traditional healers. Untrained or partly trained dentists provide oral healthcare, at least to some degree, in many cultures where HCPs are unregulated. Traditional healers in some countries, for example South Africa, give oral health advice to their patients, and many give specific toothbrush instruc-

tion. Over 50% of such healers have been found to have had patients who presented with mouth problems and up to 90% referred patients to the formal healthcare sector. Interestingly, more than 90% of such healers may be found to correctly identify gingival inflammation, dental caries and oral candidiasis from photographs.

Disparities in Oral Healthcare of Minority Groups

There can be racial differences in the receipt and effectiveness of dental services in improving oral health-related quality of life. Race has also been shown to affect the quality of HCP-patient relations, and even healthcare insurance.

Barriers to Oral Healthcare
There are clear barriers to oral healthcare in some BME communities. These include mainly:
• socioeconomics
• language
• mistrust
• fear
• culture
• denial
• concerns about dental surgery hygiene.

Many attend for emergency care only; for example, UK studies have shown that 40% of Vietnamese attended only when in pain and 30% of Bangladeshi children had never visited a dentist.

One study revealed interesting perceptions, where cost, language and mistrust proved to be the most important barriers to dental care (Table 1 -3). These trends are not exclusive to the UK.

Effects of Acculturation
There is generally a positive impact of acculturation on the oral health status of immigrants. A beneficial effect on oral hygiene indices usually follows the introduction of toothbrushes and toothpastes to communities who have been using traditional oral hygiene materials. With motivation and support, there is sustainability of use of these adjuncts to oral hygiene.

Acculturation however, does not necessarily significantly affect awareness about the risk factors and signs of oral cancer. Habits such as betel use may continue for several decades after migration. Paan (betel nut), a risk factor in

25

Table 1-3 **Perceived barriers to dental care**

Barriers	Cost of care	Language	Mistrust of dentist (perceived unnecessary treatment)	Anxiety	Hygiene	Cultural misunderstandings
Groups most expressing concern						
Bangladeshi	+	+	+			+ (preferred female staff)
Black African	+					
Black Caribbean	+			+		
Chinese	+	+		+	+	
Indian	+	+	+			
Pakistani	+	+	+		+	
Sudanese	+	+				
Turkish	+		+			
Vietnamese	+	+		+	+	

★ Adapted from Newton et al., 2001

oral submucous fibrosis and oral cancer, is commonly used among South Asian ethnic groups in the UK, but not among Sikhs (as with smoking) or Punjabis. Bangladeshis are particularly likely to retain the betel habit, significantly more females than males chewing and adding tobacco to their quid. Indian ethnic migrants to the UK appear to have a significantly higher incidence of oral and oropharyngeal cancer compared with the native UK population.

Addressing Disparities in Healthcare

Historically, many HCPs serving ethnic populations have been members of the same ethnic/racial/religious group. Other HCPs have traditionally had their own expectations of how healthcare should be provided and how patients are supposed to respond to care. If they are to work effectively with a multicultural population, HCPs, including dentists, must alter traditional approaches to treating patients.

The degree to which race, ethnicity, religion or cultural factors influence an individual's perception of a given illness and the decision to seek healthcare are important components of the healthcare access problem. For this reason, a basic knowledge of the health status and needs of the group being served is fundamental in providing culturally sensitive healthcare. Even within seemingly homogeneous environments, cultural factors affecting healthcare can be missed and the quality of the patient/HCP provider relationship is compromised.

It is imperative therefore, that all dental HCPs acquire the knowledge and communication skills that will make them attentive to the cultural differences of their patients. One of the best ways to achieve this is to work or become involved in the relevant communities.

A workforce of increasing diversity that can address the disparities in oral health problems based on race and ethnicity is also needed. The US Institute of Medicine (IOM) report entitled *Unequal Treatment: Confronting Racial and Ethnic Disparities in Healthcare* found that there are racial and ethnic disparities in healthcare and that a lack of access to care does not fully explain why such disparities exist. The IOM report showed bias, stereotyping, prejudice and clinical uncertainty as possible contributing causes and catalysed the medical profession to re-examine its institutions and training programmes in relation to cultural competence.

Affirmative action was subsequently introduced into US academic dental institutions. Life-performance questions added to the written applications to dental school are designed to assess the candidates' personal characteristics, including leadership, community service, realistic self-appraisal, personal support system, ability to deal with racism and ability to set goals and self-responsibility. This action increased the diversity of the dental student population, and will ultimately achieve a body of more diverse dental HCPs. Similar changes may follow in other countries, with anticipated improvements in culturally sensitive healthcare.

Addressing Disparities in Oral Health
Efforts to address disparities in oral health include public education and community screening efforts, dental curriculum development, professional education, intensive research efforts, together with oral health education/awareness programme. These programmes may be customized to HCPs and HCP trainees and to populations at risk. Previous difficulties in addressing disparities in oral health are considered to highlight the changing nature of the challenge, let alone its increasing complexity.

Culturally Sensitive Healthcare

Culturally sensitive healthcare should:
• provide respectful care
• meet the patient's personal, religious and cultural needs
• educate and inform on health issues
• enable patients to make their own choices
• respect those choices.

Culturally sensitive healthcare is impossible without knowledge about cultural and ethnic issues, but the simple acquisition of such knowledge is not enough, as attitudes and skills must also be developed. It is important to recognise and respect the uniqueness and dignity of each individual patient, and to respond appropriately to their need for care, irrespective of their religion, ethnic origin, gender, sexual preferences, personal attributes, nature of their health problem or any other factor.

Stereotyping comes from jumping to conclusions based on insufficient data; the skill is to determine where generalisation ends and stereotyping begins. Stereotyped attitudes towards religious, ethnic or cultural groups are common, both from the majority group towards the minority, and vice versa. In some instances, religious and cultural identities overlap significantly, as in the case of Muslims and Arabs but – while most Arabs are Muslim, by no means are all Muslims Arabs. In many instances, religion has a stronger effect on culture than do other factors. It is crucial to remember, however, that there is considerable variation in every cultural group and therefore the only way to provide high-quality and culturally sensitive care is to listen sensitively to each person, and ask them, when appropriate, about their needs and wishes.

Cultures – Recognising without Stereotyping

The dentist and dental care professionals (DCP – therapist, hygienists etc) must be aware of the possibility that their patient may be from another culture. In some instances this is easy, if the dentist or DCP has advance notice or reviews the records of booked patients - for example from the patient's title, e.g. 'Father', indicating he is probably a Roman Catholic priest. There are also many indications of a culture, of varying utility. Some of these indications may provide fairly hard evidence of another culture, including:

• language
• writing
• clothing
• jewellery and amulets.

It is crucially important, however, to avoid jumping to conclusions or stereotyping. For example, it is important not to guess patient's ethnicity and/or religion from their appearance, dress and any insignia that they may be wearing. With this important caveat, it can, however, be helpful to consider key indicators.

Language: it may be immediately obvious that the patients speaks another language, or speaks the local language poorly with a detectable foreign accent or atypical word formation, with lack of understanding of various expressions. Alternatively, the patient may use a form of greeting that gives a clue to their origins.

Writing: it may be apparent that the patient's written communication is from another culture. This may take the form of poor use of local language or unusual phraseology that may give a clue to their origins.

Clothing: while most Anglo-Americans wear suits on occasion, suits are not the prerogative of any culture. Neither are the kameez or sari typically worn by South Asians. In contrast, clothing such as the Arab 'dishdash', the Muslim 'purdah' or shawl and headcap 'tigiyah', the Sikh 'turban' and the Jewish male cap 'kippah' and female wig 'sheitel' are so distinctive as to virtually guarantee accurate identification of the culture.

Jewellery and amulets: in some cultures, clearly visible amulets (protective devices worn around the body, or placed next to other objects to protect individuals from various evils) or jewellery may be worn, such as a necklace with the Christian cross, St. Christopher pendant, or the Jewish Mager David. The Hindu 'mangalsutra' of married women or the wrist threads worn by men may be less well known.

Other visible signs can provide far less robust evidence, including:
• hair and/or moustache/beard style
• facial and other appearance
• behaviour
• diet
• habits
• homes and families
• names.

Jumping to wrong conclusions, although a well-intentioned attempt at cultural sensitivity, may cause offence and loss of confidence in you by the patient. If you are quick to form opinions on limited evidence and get things wrong, how reliable are you in diagnosing disease?

Hair and/or moustache/beard style: the 'dreadlocks' of the Rastafarian are obvious, but not restricted to people of that faith. The beard and uncut hair of Sikhs is fairly distinctive. The hairstyle of Orthodox Jews is also fairly distinctive. Many Muslims retain a beard, but not all. Many people have hair of different length or a shaved head, a particular hairstyle, or beard or moustache of a certain form unrelated to any special religious or cultural background and may be troubled, if not annoyed, if such things were considered indicative of culture or religious belief.

Facial and other appearance: facial appearance and skin and eye colour can be a good guide to ancestry, but not necessarily religion or culture. Marks on the forehead to signify marriage are seen in many Hindus ('kukum') and Sikhs ('bindi') but not all. Tattoos may be distinctive. The forearm tattoo used by Nazi Germans to brand Jews and others in the 1930s–40s is probably distinctive, but other tattoos of a decorative nature may simply have been adopted.

Behaviour: This is a very tenuous way to attempt to identify a culture. Habits, however, such as bowing are more common in Asian than other cultures, as is the preferred use of chopsticks.

Diet: People vary widely within cultures in their diet – diets in general in multiracial societies having become very diverse. Some elements of a diet may, however, be indicative of culture or possibly religious belief. For example, snails are rarely eaten outside France, guinea pig is enjoyed by Peruvians, but rarely eaten elsewhere, and certain types of bread may be limited to a religious faith. In addition, items excluded from a diet, for example pork or shellfish, may be a strong indication of a culture or belief.

Habits: Chewing gum is common in Anglo-American cultures, but in Asian cultures the chewing of tobacco or betel is common.

Homes and families: This is again a tenuous way to identify someone from a culture, but there are areas inhabited exclusively or largely by particular cultures.

Names: names can be misleading, increasingly so with acculturation. Indeed, some people change their names – this was commonplace for example, in Jewish German, Polish, Russian and other immigrant peoples entering the UK before the Second World War. In other cases, names can be indicative of religions or cultures: for example, most people with the first name 'Mohammad' are Muslim, as are most people with Arabic last names such as 'El-Kabbir'. Men's names such as Bhai, Chand, Das, Dev, Kant, Kumar, Lal, Nat, Pal, or women's names such as Behn, Devi, Gowri, Kumari, Lakshmi, Rani or a family name such as Patel are commonly Hindu. Sikh identity is shown by the male name Singh or female Kaur.

Less visible signs of a culture can include:
• reactions to events
• norms
• values
• concepts of right and wrong
• orientation towards time
• occupation rarely (Rabbis are invariably Jews and Imams are Muslims).

However, we stress again that it is important not to guess patient's ethnicity and/or religion from their appearance, dress and any insignia that they may be wearing – ie, not to fall into the inappropriate practice of stereotyping.

To overcome the difficulties of challenging patients as to their ethnicity and/or religious beliefs, we suggest fostering a culture in clinical situations whereby patients respond to clinicians' wishes to be culturally sensitive in their provision of care by volunteering information about their ethnicity/religious beliefs they wish taken into consideration in their treatment. Arrangements to foster such a culture may include statements in patient information leaflets, posters/notices in patient waiting areas, and the inclusion of an explanation of the goal of culturally sensitive care in websites intended for patients. There may be value in having such information in various languages according to geographic location and patient population.

In encouraging patients to volunteer information about their ethnicity and religious faith, it is important to stress that knowledge of such information will in no way influence the quality of care and, of course, that any disclosures will be treated in strictest confidence, together with all other personal data.

In hospital environments in which patients may have previously given information on ethnicity and their religious faith as part of, for example, an inpatient admission procedure, clinicians should make a special point of looking for and noting this information and, if appropriate/necessary, confirming the details with the patient. Such confirmation may be best achieved by, for example, an indirect question or statement such as 'I note that you are ...'. Such provisions may also apply in other clinical environments, including a culturally sensitive general practice, when, for example, a new member of the dental team sees a regular-attending patient for the first time.

Other considerations could include recruiting the support of local community/religious leaders to encourage people to volunteer information to HCPs to help promote culturally sensitive healthcare provision. Additional drivers could come through community campaigns to have patients and HCPs work together to develop healthcare provision appropriate for a multicultural population.

In terms of health and healthcare, cultures often differ in beliefs and attitudes about:
• what is regarded as health
• what is considered to cause illness
• how symptoms are perceived
• what is regarded as good healthcare
• attitudes towards traditional medicines and treatments
• attitudes towards western healing, HCPs and medicines.

Clearly the management of a patient who believes that their illness is the result of an evil influence or failure to conform to some practice or tradition should be different to the management of a patient who does not have such views. Understanding why patients believe they are ill and their views on possible remedies can be very important in achieving a satisfactory clinical outcome.

Healthcare Values in Different Cultures

Historically, throughout the world, illness has variously been attributed to witchcraft, demons or the will of god(s). These concepts still retain some power, both in the developing world and in some westernised societies, where faithhealing is still common. Traditional healing and alternative medicines are used increasingly in cultures, in parallel with moves against, for example, genetically modified (GM) foods and other 'engineered' products.

Anglo-American values of the majority cultures in the western world significantly affect healthcare and the behavior of HCPs, and can be summarised by beliefs in:
* individualism
* informed consent
* science and technology
* separation of health from spiritual health.
* orientation towards clock time.

Thus, according to Anglo-American (westernised) values, the body is partitioned into organs and systems, each with identifiable functions, and is seen as functioning well unless disrupted by disease.

Westernised medicine has advanced health more through improvements in public health and nutrition than through medicine itself, albeit that advances in pharmacology, surgery, medical technology and related health sciences in and since the 20th century have made great strides. With the advent of evidence-based medicine, the process of change is set to continue. Modern westernised medicine, despite the hypochondria of western society and the increasing focus on form rather than function, is uniquely effective and widespread compared with traditional healing. Life is paced according to clock time, which continues to be valued more than personal or subjective time.

The westernised patient rarely expects the HCP to have all the answers or make all the decisions and, increasingly, expects a healthcare partnership with the HCP. As a result, the patient increasingly takes a role by asking questions and discussing the diagnosis and treatment recommendations with the HCP. No longer is medical or dental advice accepted without question. The nature of modern medicine has also spawned considerable social disquiet, as evinced by concerns about doctors' and scientists' motives and professionalism. The capabilities of modern medicine, however, have done little to improve the lot of the developing world. Indeed, it is clear that westernisation has had a significant negative impact on some cultures: for example, a dietary change to refined carbohydrates has been associated with dental caries, obesity and other problems. Not to mention the effect of globalisation on the environment and transmission of infections.

Non-Anglo-American cultures may view health and disease and healthcare in a strikingly different fashion. Indeed, entire systems of healing are built upon indigenous beliefs and traditions, with patients possibly holding very different understandings of health and disease. In terms of oral healthcare patients may hold traditional views of health and disease. Some patients may, due to cultural or historical experiences, expect tooth conservation, but others may expect extraction. High prices or lack of access to treatment may lead to neglect of dental care, where this is not seen as a priority.

In such cultures, the patient may expect the HCP to have all the answers and make all the decisions. As a result, the patient often takes a passive role, answering but not asking questions, and waiting for the HCP to impart the diagnosis and recommendations. Most of the time medical or dental advice is accepted without question. Patients may regard as sensitive issues matters that are sometimes more freely discussed by westernised patients. Head-nodding and smiles do not always signify comprehension or agreement; some patients are reluctant to disagree with HCPs.

If western treatment fails to bring immediate relief of the symptoms, certain patients may seek the care of a traditional physician or healer. The same thing may happen if a western diagnosis is rejected because it bears a negative prognosis (including diagnosis of a long-term illness or of an illness that cannot be fully cured) or because surgery is advised. The traditional treatment may either replace the western treatment or be used along with it. However, many patients do not disclose the use of traditional care and medications to their western HCPs because the two medical domains – western and traditional medicine – are seen as separate. Patients from some cultures may also fear that the western HCP (an authority figure) will disapprove, or they believe that disclosure of the traditional care would violate the relationship of trust. Some patients may wish to bring gifts to the HCP and can be insulted by an ill-considered response, let alone rejection.

In treating non-Anglo-American patients in developed countries, HCPs should guard against assuming that they express feelings and reactions in the same way that Anglo-American patients do. For example, Anglo-Americans, in general, are taught to be stoic and not to cry out in pain unless the discomfort is extreme. To do otherwise is considered self-indulgent or childish. But many non-Anglo-Americans are taught that the proper way to handle pain is to let it out vocally. Another example is found in decision-making by women concerning their healthcare: Anglo-American providers may fail to understand women who, according to their custom, delegate the decisions to their husbands. Furthermore, some men find it difficult to accept the opinion of a female HCP.

Cultural Assessment
It is critical that HCPs are able to assess and understand cultural differences and learn to communicate across cultural divides. Respect and communication between the HCP and patient, and time, are fundamental to success. Given that there is considerable variation in every cultural group, the only way to provide culturally sensitive care is to listen sensitively to each person, and ask them, when appropriate, about their background, needs and wishes. This requires time, patience and expertise.

Pertinent questions may seek information in respect of:
- preferred name
- ethnic affiliation, and its strength
- place of birth
- time spent in the host country
- preferred language in which to communicate and level of understanding of the language of the host country
- religious beliefs, and their importance in daily life
- education
- occupation
- economic circumstances
- how the patient considers they relate or differ from their cultural group
- support from family and friends; availability and strength
- food habits, preferences and restrictions
- health/illness beliefs and practices.

Great care and sensitivity is required in phrasing and putting such questions,

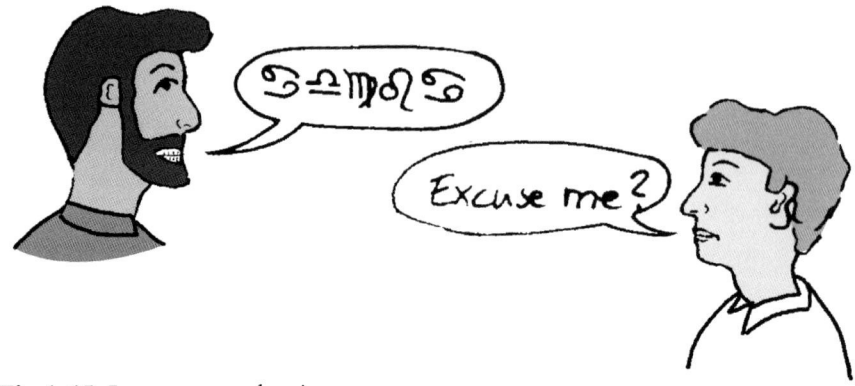

Fig 1-15 Language as a barrier.

as there is the risk of causing offence and mistrust. This may be reduced by pre-empting at least the more contentious questions with an explanation of the need to obtain certain information.

Clinicians must remember how cultural health practices influence:
• the patient's knowledge of the illness
• the role of the family in decision-making
• the perceived role of dentists and other staff
• the trust in oral healthcare providers of different cultures
• the role of traditional or faith healers, or remedies.

Remember that not all cultures value time or punctuality as do some Anglo-Americans. Some have other values: involvement with people and completion of interpersonal encounters is more valued than 'being on time'.

Communicating
Communicating requires time, patience and expertise: language can be a huge barrier (Fig 1-15). One of the most obvious ways to assist communication is to have clinic and other signs and material available in relevant languages (Figs 1-16, 1-17).

Patient interviews are an opportunity to listen and assess important aspects of the patient and his/her situation, feelings and concerns about healthcare. The history offers the opportunity to explore with the patient what beliefs and practices are important to them. Patients are the experts on their lives, cultures and experiences and, if asked with respect and sensitivity, they will usually tell the HCP how best to provide care for them.

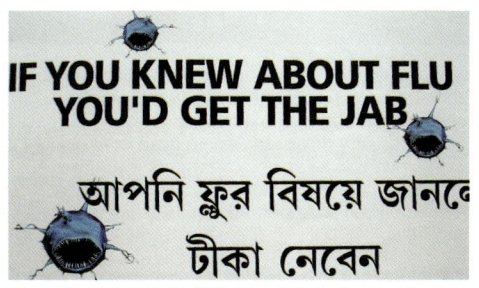

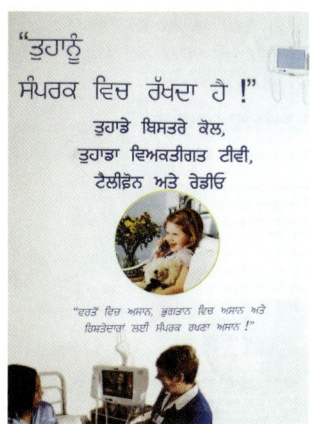

Figs 1-16 and 1-17 Health information for a multicultural population.

Communicating across a language and/or cultural barrier can be time-consuming, difficult and frustrating. It is important, therefore, to:

- provide an environment conducive to carrying out effective history taking. Privacy and confidentiality are important if not crucial, so try and minimise non-essential people in the room unless the patients needs or wants family, friends or an interpreter present.
- ask patients about their preferred language. HCPs must learn to recognise those patient interactions where an interpreter will minimise or eliminate any communication and cultural barriers between them and the patient.
- use direct eye contact, even if avoided by patient, and speak slowly and clearly, using uncomplicated terminology, remembering that some individuals have hearing impairment.
- remember that even those with a good grasp of the language may not necessarily understand medical or dental terminology. Explain as you go along.
- remember that head-nodding and smiles do not necessarily indicate understanding or agreement. Ask questions to ascertain understanding, not just enquiries with a 'yes' or 'no' answer. Silence can have many meanings and sometimes indicates lack of agreement.
- never assume agreement or fluency until you are sure from the feedback from the patient. Remember that oral fluency in a language often exceeds skills in reading and writing. Do not get disturbed if a bilingual patient reverts to their native tongue to speak with family or friends, as they are almost certainly not gossiping.

- establish who is the spokesperson for the patient and the patient's confidence in that person, if the patient wishes others to speak for them.

Greeting Patients
Greetings can 'make' or 'break' the professional relationship with a patient. Key points to remember include:
- smile
- speak clearly and directly to the patient, making eye contact as appropriate
- greet using 'Good morning' or 'Good afternoon', or the greeting appropriate to the culture concerned (see below: ensuring you are correct!)
- never use the personal (first) name alone, except for children and when requested. Ask the patient for their family name and the most used personal name, and use title and surname, confirming pronunciation if uncertain.
- be careful about touching (see below)
- explain who you are and what you do, what is happening and what will happen
- sensitively enquire as to whether the patient understands the conversation
- if possible, say a few words in the person's language or say something to put the patient at ease.
- encourage the patient to establish a relationship.

Different cultures and religions have different traditions in greetings (Table 1-4). For many people, the customary greeting is a gesture other than the handshake. In addition, some may be uncomfortable shaking hands with a person of the opposite sex. For many, this may not be an issue at all, while for others it may create challenges.

Unless you are certain of their culture or religion, it is often best to greet a patient with a handshake, assuming the patient, in particular a woman offers her hand, and then say 'Good morning/afternoon' and use their given title (Mr, Mrs, Miss, Dr, etc.) followed by their family or surname name.

Notions of Modesty
Many cultures have rules or concepts about clothing to be worn, about what areas of the body can be exposed, and about touching and personal space.
- Virtually all patients can be embarrassed by feeling exposed, in particular to the gaze of strangers or people of the opposite gender. Patients should not be embarrassed.
- Do not remove clothing, head coverings, amulets or jewellery unnecessarily. If such items must be removed, place them carefully in a clean receptacle on a raised surface.

Table 1-4 **Greeting patients of different cultures and religions**

Culture or religion	Physical greeting	Verbal greeting
Africans	Greet with a handshake.	Use their title (Mr, Mrs, Miss, Dr, etc.) followed by their last name and say 'Good morning/afternoon'.
Americans (North)	Greet with a handshake.	Use their title followed by their last name and say 'Good morning/afternoon'.
Americans (South)	Greet with a handshake.	Use their title followed by their first or last name and say 'Good morning/afternoon'.
Arabs	Greet men with a handshake. To avoid any offence, it is safer to wait to see if a woman wishes to shake hands.	Use their title followed by their last name and say 'As Salamu Alaiakum'. In the Middle East, Arabs prefer the use of titles e.g. Dr, or to be called Abu (father of) the name of the first born child, e.g. Abu Faisal (father of Faisal).
Australasians	Greet with a handshake.	Use their title followed by their last name and say 'Good morning/afternoon/day'.
Buddhists	Lay Buddhists are no different from other lay people. Bowing is a common practice in Asia, both within and outside religious circles –	Use their title followed by their last name and say 'Good morning/afternoon'.

Culture or religion	Physical greeting	Verbal greeting
	a way of expressing respect and reverence, as well as a form of greeting. Greet Buddhist monks and nuns with a small bow with hands together in front of the chest and avoid hand-shaking.	
Caribbeans	Greet with a handshake.	Use their title followed by their last name and say 'Good morning/afternoon'.
Central Asians	Bowing is a common practice. Greet with a slight bow and a handshake. Shake hands with a woman only if she offers hers.	Use their title followed by their first or last name and say 'Good morning/ afternoon'.
Chinese	Bowing is a common practice. Greet with a slight bow and a handshake. Shake hands with woman only if she offers hers.	Use their title followed by their last name and say 'Good morning/afternoon'.
Christians	Greet with a handshake. In some cultures, such as those of southern Europe, people known to each other may greet by touching cheek to cheek.	Use their title followed by their last name and say 'Good morning/afternoon'.
Europeans	Greet with a handshake.	Greet the patient using their title followed by their last name.

Culture or religion	Physical greeting	Verbal greeting
Hindus	Greet with a handshake. Whenever a Hindu meets a Hindu, they greet with hands together at chin level.	Use their title followed by their last name and say 'Namaste' or 'Jai Swaminarayan'.
Jains	Greet only men with a handshake. Whenever a Jain meets a Jain, they place hands together at chin level, and bow.	Use their title followed by their last name and say 'Jai Jinendra'.
Jews	Greet men with a handshake. To avoid any offence, it is prudent to wait to see if a woman wishes to shake hands.	Use their title followed by their first and last names. The Jewish naming system follows the international convention of first names and a surname although Jews also have a Hebrew name for use in synagogue and on religious documents.
Muslims	Greet men with a handshake. To avoid any offence, it is prudent to wait to see if a woman wishes to shake hands.	Use their title followed by their first and last names and say 'As Salamu Alaiakum' (May peace be with you). The naming system used depends on the area from which the Muslim comes.
Roma	Greet with a handshake. Whenever a Roma meets another Roma, they greet each other with a raised palm.	Use their title followed by their last name and say 'Good morning/afternoon' or the words in Roma for luck and health 'baxt hai sastimos'.

Culture or religion	Physical greeting	Verbal greeting
Sikhs	Greet men with a handshake. To avoid offence, it is prudent to wait to see if a woman wishes to shake hands. Whenever a Sikh meets another Sikh, they greet each other with folded hands.	Use their title followed by their first and last names and say 'Waheguru Ji Ka Khalsa, Waheguru Ji Ki Fateh' or less formally 'Sat Sri Akal'.
South Asians	Unless you are aware they are Hindu or Muslim (then see above), bowing is a common practice. Greet with a slight bow and a handshake. Shake hands with a woman only if she offers hers.	Use their title followed by their first or last name and say 'Good morning/ afternoon'.
South East Asians	Unless you are aware they are Hindu or Muslim (then see above), bowing is a common practice. Greet with a slight bow and a handshake. Shake hands with a woman only if she offers hers.	Use their title followed by their first or last name and say 'Good morning/ afternoon'.

- Establish the patient's concerns, if any, about opposite gender HCPs and try to comply. Always have a chaperone present, preferably of the same gender as the patient.
- Ensure appropriate facilities for washing are available (see *Facilities*).

Touching Patients
- volunteer your right hand to shake the right hand with a male patient
- do not shake hands with a female patient unless she offers her hand first

- keep a respectful distance
- touch within gender only; take care to touch only hands or upper limbs, not the head or other parts of the body. Particular care is necessary when treating patients in a supine position.
- give things with your right hand only, even if left-handed. In some cultures, both hand are used, but do not assume this to be the case.

Interpreting
Language barriers are the most difficult to overcome. Certain situations may necessitate the use of an interpreter. In preference, in many cultures try not to use family members, or interpreters/advocates of different sects, since there may be:
- role conflicts
- lack of medical vocabulary or understanding
- confused perceptions or misunderstandings
- withholding or distorting of information
- differences in health beliefs
- potential for conflict (e.g. between Turks and Kurds).

However, in some cultures and with some individuals there can be concern and mistrust if the patient believes the interpreter may not accurately convey their messages to the HCP. In these circumstances, the patient may prefer a family member or friend to an acquaintance as interpreter. Failing that, a professional interpreter may be required.

Where indicated, use interpreters of the same gender as the patient, preferably no younger than the patient, and not from any sect/religion/tribe that might be unacceptable – always ensuring first that the patient is comfortable with the interpreter. They should therefore meet, before the interview, which also allows the interpreter also to assess the patient. It is crucial before proceeding to take the history, to:
- tell the interpreter exactly what you want to achieve
- ask the interpreter not to omit or insert information
- allocate adequate time
- speak in short units of speech
- check the interpreter's understanding.

Taking a Culturally Sensitive History
History taking requires time, patience and expertise. Apart from considerable care to deal tactfully with cultural and religious issues should they arise, and maintaining confidentiality, other do's and do nots are shown in Table 1-5.

Table 1-5 **Culturally sensitive communications**

DOs	DO NOTs
Smile	Smile at inopportune times, as this may be interpreted as lack of respect and under-standing
Say a few words of interest about the patient's background	Appear disinterested in the patient's back-ground
Act calmly	Be dismissive, aggressive or threatening
Speak clearly and slowly	Speak too loud, too fast or raise voice
Sit at same level as patient	Sit with the legs crossed, lean on a table or desk, or point at anything with the foot when talking
Maintain personal space	Touch the patient unless so invited, or offer anything with the left hand
Look at patient	Point
Establish eye contact	Challenge or argue
Satisfy yourself that the patient hears and understands you	Assume fluency or agreement, or let frustration show in your approach
Listen to patient	Joke
Look attentive	Trivialise
Give time	Interrupt
Behave in a sympathetic manner	Change subject
Remember people understand much more than they express	Offer platitudes

DOs	DO NOTs
Use short sentences	Ask sensitive questions. If you need to, use same gender family member as advocate.
	Patients may be sensitive to questions about sexuality and emotional problems.
	There may be stigma about illness, cancer, congenital and genetic diseases, drug abuse and infections such as HIV, TB, leprosy or STIs.
Use uncomplicated language	Avoid the use of: • technical terms and expressions • abbreviations • professional jargon • abstract concepts • colloquialisms • idiomatics • slang • metaphors • euphemisms • stereotype figures or symbols
Be encouraging and honest	Assume an individual's beliefs and practices regarding healthcare
Observe reactions carefully	Be judgmental, based on personal beliefs
Summarize, so that patient can indicate their understanding, or help you understand better	Conclude with unnecessarily complex explanations and lack of clarity over the way forward.
If in doubt, check the under-	Attempt to remove any clothing, necklace, bracelet standing of the patient or other item that might have religious or cultural significance

DOs	DO NOTs
Give any bad or unpleasant news tactfully and slowly	Give any bad or unpleasant news too quickly
Maintain confidentiality and check with the patient exactly who can be told about their condition, when, and what they can be told	Talk with friends or others about the patient, unless so instructed

Sensitive Issues in the History
Considerable thought and care should be taken when considering discussing sensitive topics, such as matters relating to:
• sexual matters
  – personal relationships
  – marital matters
  – reproductive issues
• communicable infections, in particular
  – HIV/AIDS
  – sexually transmitted infections
  – tuberculosis
  – leprosy
• mental and psychological health problems
• cancer and other potentially lethal disease
• genetic problems
• financial matters and socioeconomic status.

These should never be discussed with children or strangers and, unless the patient agrees, not with friends or family or persons (including interpreters) of the opposite sex.

Examination
An examination requires time, a systematic, patient approach and clinical skill. Key considerations include:
• Value modesty and privacy. It is best to close doors and take steps to avoid people seeing through windows. Have as few people around as possible. Expose only those parts of the body necessary for the examination.
• Always have a chaperone present, even with a same-gender patient.

- Always consider, especially when the chaperone is of opposite gender, whether the patient is content with the chaperone.
- Give careful consideration to the arrangements to have, where necessary, any other accompanying person or interpreter attend the examination.
- Observe reactions carefully, in particular embarrassment, unease and suspicion.
- Check understanding and consent. The law on consent applies to individuals from other countries, no different to other members of the public, but they may not know this. Where appropriate, it can be wise to involve family members in the process, but not as interpreters.
- Remember that silence can have various meanings, sometimes disagreement.
- Remember people understand much more than they speak, not least from facial expressions and other non-verbal clues.

Investigations, Therapy and Prognostication
- Never assume that you can predict the acceptability of interventions and related treatment based on generalisations. Always ascertain the individual's beliefs and practices regarding healthcare.
- Illustrate a point with diagrams, models or pictures. However, avoid the use of stereotype figures and symbols (which may offend Muslims and some others).
- Take care to communicate carefully any bad or difficult news to patients and, where appropriate, family and accompanying persons.
- Remember that the patient or family may, in some cultures, view illness as 'God's will' or, alternatively, some form of retribution.
- Do not dismiss the possible complementary use of traditional or herbal medicine or remedies.
- Explain the need for written consent and related documentation. In obtaining consent, patients must understand what the proposed procedures involve and the possible adverse consequences. Also explain, as necessary, that there are legal requirements to obtain consent.
- Instruct drug use as a dose given every 'n' hours, rather than advise 'n' times daily.
- Wherever possible, avoid treatment on main religious holidays or periods of fasting.
- Avoid touching or cutting hair or shaving an area without express consent.
- Treat all patient information as confidential. Check that the patient is prepared to have information provided to other HCPs, or to the family.
- Give continuity of care.
In proceeding to investigations and subsequent treatment, it is considered

important to have developed a profile of the patient's religious and ethnic background and beliefs. To be able to do this effectively, it is important to have knowledge of the outlining features of various religions and ethnic groups, as set out in the following sections of this book, and to have ascertained the extent to which the individual patient subscribes to relevant beliefs, traditions, practices and taboos.

Patient Information
Patient information can be useful if visual or oral, or written in a language and style patients can readily understand. Such information should be:
• pertinent
• immediately relevant
• sensitive to the values, way of life and knowledge of the patient
• non-patronising
• respectful
• helpful.

Avoid the use of stereotype figures and symbols (which may cause offence to some).

Concerns about Healthcare Products
Concerns regarding the use of animal products in healthcare provision are widespread and problematical. Others are concerned about the use of alcohol. Some key specific concerns for different groups of patients are set out in Table 1-6. Individuals may share concerns with people in other groups. These often relate to the use of animal-derived healthcare products or, for inpatients, various dietary constituents. Stereotyping must be avoided in managing individual patients.

Eating pork is proscribed in certain faiths, as is the prescribing, administration and taking of porcine-derived medicines or other healthcare products.
• Judaism and Islam in particular strictly forbid porcine products.
• Buddhism, Hinduism and Sikhism see vegetarianism as a sign of spirituality. Pork is not eaten and porcine products are best avoided. Some patients, particularly those who follow vegan or vegetarian diets, may object to the use of animals to meet the needs of humans.
• Christians, especially in Afro-Caribbean communities, and Rastafarians may choose not to eat pork, despite there being no dietary restriction.

As a consequence, many modern healthcare products have replaced animal-

Table 1-6 **Key dietary concerns for certain groups of patients**

Groups	Key concerns
Buddhists	Animal and genetically modified (GM) products
Christians	Use of healthcare products and consumables produced through exploitation of disadvantaged people. Animal products, if production has involved cruelty to animals or animal research
Catholics	GM derivatives and those developed by fetal experimentation
Jehovah's witnesses	Not able to accept food and products that may contain blood or blood derivatives
Hindus	Gelatin-containing products, animal products and alcohol
Jains	Strict vegetarians, but will not eat root vegetables. Some patients, in particular those who follow vegan or vegetarian diets, may object to the use of animals to meet the needs of humans
Muslims	Porcine and bovine derivatives, alcohol, non-Halal animal derivatives, E numbers derived from porcine products, and emulsifiers derived from animals
Jews	Shellfish and products derived not only from pork, but also from any animal not slaughtered according to Jewish law (Kosher). Devout Jews may wish to avoid alcohol
Sikhs	Beef and its derivatives

and human-derived medicines and related items, and are to be preferred because they:
- reduce the potential risk of biological contamination
- have specificity, predictable activity, interbatch consistency and unlimited sourcing
- are useful clinical alternatives for those with a religious or cultural objection to animal and human derived products (e.g. vegan, vegetarians).

Commonly Used Agents of Animal Derivation
Gelatin and lactose, obtained from bovine sources, found as exipients in some products may be unacceptable to some faiths such as Hindus. There is also some concern that gelatin might have been obtained from cows with bovine spongiform encephalopathy (BSE) and may thus pose a risk to humans. Gelatin is made of protein derived from animal bones, cartilage, tendons and other tissues such as pig skin. Isinglass, used in the manufacture of some alcoholic drinks, is a type of gelatin from the air bladders of certain kinds of fish. Aspic is made from clarified meat, fish or vegetable stocks and gelatin.

Haemostatic Agents
Blood and blood products such as blood clotting factors were, in the past, typically derived from human or animal material. Recombinant factors are now widely available, avoiding the religious objections (e.g. amongst Jehovah's witnesses) and also potential risks of transmission of infections (e.g. HIV, hepatitis B virus, hepatitis C virus, prions, etc.).

Topical haemostatic agents may, however, still be obtained from an animal source, as shown in Table 1-7, and may thus be contraindicated in some patients on cultural/religious grounds - unless they are of synthetic origin.

Establishing if a Drug is of Animal Origin
- Check the drug name - porcine may be written on the label
- Check the *Summary of Product Characteristics*
- Contact the manufacturer and ask their medicines information department for specific detail of the origin of the drug
- Check the Patient Information Leaflet – but this does not always detail all the components.

Oral Healthcare Products that may Contain Culturally Unacceptable Materials
The dental HCP must also be aware of problems posed by certain dental materials and consumables. However, some religions, though apparently

Table 1-7 **Some topical haemostatic agents**

Agent	Main constituent	Origin
Avitene	Collagen	Bovine
Colla-Cote	Collagen	Bovine
Gelfoam	Gelatin	Bovine
Helistat	Collagen	Bovine
Instat	Collagen	Bovine
Thrombinar	Thrombin	Bovine
Thrombogen	Thrombin	Bovine
Thrombostat	Thrombin	Bovine
Beriplast	Fibrin	Various
Cyclokapron	Tranexamic acid	Synthetic
Surgicel	Cellulose	Synthetic

objecting to some constituents, do not actually bar their use if the product is designed to enhance health.

Some oral healthcare products are licensed as pharmacological products and must, as a consequence, be labelled with all ingredients – active and inactive. This readily affords the opportunity to avoid certain religious and ethnic group restrictions. Examples include products such as Corsodyl (chlorhexidine) mouthwash, which are acceptable to all groups.

Most oral healthcare products are licensed only as 'cosmetics', which are less rigorously tested than pharmacological products, although they must still be labelled with all active and inactive ingredients. Most toothpastes fall into this category.

Table 1-8 **Examples of alcohol-containing and alcohol-free mouthwashes**

Alcohol-containing products	% alcohol v/v	Alcohol-free products
Listermint	13	Oral B Anti-Plaque Dental Rinse Alcohol Free
Listerine Mouthwash	26.9	RetarDEX oral spray and oral rinse
Scope Mouthwash	19	Colgate rinse alcohol-free
Search	15.3	TheraBreath
Mentadent Mouthwash	12	Dentyl pH
Oral B Dental Rinse	9.4	Macleans Alcohol Free Smoothmint Mouthwash
Colgate Fluorigard Daily	4.96	Yotuel Whitening Mouthwash
Macleans Active Mouthguard	17.5	Frador coolmint mouth-wash

Notwithstanding these rules, it is often difficult to ascertain exactly what is in oral healthcare products and certain dental materials and related consumables. This can be problematic since some contain animal products, or agents such as alcohol (ethanol) that might not be acceptable to members of certain religions and cultures. Furthermore, the same product may be in one country labelled as containing for example, gelatin, but that fact may be omitted in another country.

Product data sheets listing all ingredients should be available for all licensed products from the original manufacturer, but they can appear incomplete.

Mouthwashes
The ingredients of mouthwashes vary. Some contain colourants or excipients

that may be animal derivatives and many contain alcohol, which may raise objections on religious grounds – although the objections are not always well-founded, when the religious rules are consulted (see Islam). Examples of alcohol-containing and alcohol-free mouthwashes are given in Table 1-8.

Dentifrices (toothpastes)
Toothpastes usually contain:
- fluoride (sodium monofluorophosphate/ amine fluoride/stannous fluoride)
- colourant
- flavouring
- foaming agents
- detergents
- humectants (prevent the paste from hardening)
- various other agents (e.g. triclosan/ polyvinylmethylether/maleic acid copolymer; sodium lauryl sulfate (SLS); potassium nitrate; potassium citrate; zinc citrate; zinc citrate trihydrate; betaine; tetrasodium pyrophosphate; tetrapotassium pyrophosphate; polypyrophosphate; essential oils).

Whitening dentifrices may contain:
- sodium hexametaphosphate (polypyrophosphate)
- sodium tripolyphosphate
- hydrogen peroxide.

Herbal toothpastes may contain:
- peppermint oil
- myrrh
- plant extract (e.g. strawberry extract)
- sanguinarine
- special oils and cleansing agents.

Not all of the ingredients of all toothpastes are clear from the labelling. Some toothpaste may also contain 'glycerin', manufactured synthetically or derived from animal fat, and this may not be included in the ingredients. Such toothpastes may be contraindicated for use on religious or cultural grounds.

Artificial salivas
Some artificial saliva preparations contain animal mucin (such as in Saliva Orthana) which may be unacceptable on religious grounds to some Muslims, Hindus, Jews and Rastafarians. Products containing carboxymethylcellulose (e.g. Glandosane or Luborant) may be preferred by some individuals.

Other products that might contain animal derivatives
Oral healthcare products that might contain animal derivatives could include
some:
- alginates
- analgesics
- antimicrobials
- bone morphogenic proteins
- bone fillers
- colourants
- drug capsules
- emulsifiers
- haemostatic materials
- mouthwashes
- periodontal membranes
- polishing (bristle) brushes
- prophylaxis pastes
- saliva replacements
- toothpastes
- waxes.

Product data sheets should be checked, in particular the data sheets for the
following materials (bovine materials are also a concern because of consid-
erations about prions – though there is no evidence of infection):
- Bovine collagen-containing products
  - Anorganic bovine bone matrix (i.e. Bio-oss)
  - Artefill (collagen/polymethylmethacrylate)
  - Bovine-derived bone morphogenic proteins
  - Bovine Graft and Bicon Resorbable Collagen Membrane
  - Bovine matrix used in OsteoGraf®/N (ABM) and PepGen P-15 (ABM
  + P-15).
  - Catgut sutures - were obtained from firmly twisted strand of intestinal
  submucosal of sheep or cattle. The supply to the UK has been stopped, and
  catgut sutures been taken off the market in France, Germany, Spain, Aus-
  tria and Japan, albeit that there is no evidence of any health risk.
  - FascianTM - a preparation of human fascia
  - Zyderm
  - Zyplast.
- Bovin gelatin-containing products
  - Chlorhexidine as a gelatin-filled chip (Perio-Chip) –
  - Crosslinked gelatin tissue adhesive (GRF ; gelatin-resorcinol mixture
  crosslinked with formaldehyde)

- Gelatin sponge (Gelfoam®)
- Gelatin-dialdehyde (GR-DIAL) (Gluetiss®)
- Hydroxyapatite -gelatin (HAP-GEL) nanocomposite
- Medijel pastilles
- Nystatin (Nystan pastilles)
- Orabase
- Resorbable gelatin sponge (Spongostan)
- Restorative material applied to the tooth surface in gelatin capsules
- Rizatriptan
- Temazepam: soft gelatin capsule formulation
- Triamcinolone acetonide in oral paste (Adcortyl in Orabase)
- Ubidicarenone (Coenzyme Q10) Gelatine Troche.
• Bovine lactose-containing products
- Endekay sodium fluoride Fluotabs 6+
- Endekay sodium fluoride mouthwash.
• Porcine materials
- BIO-GIDE Porcine collagen I & III
- Collagen membranes of porcine origin
- EMDOGAIN - derived from porcine developing enamel matrix
- Hydrocolloid Dressing with Lyophilised Porcine Dermal Skin
- Porcine bone
- Porcine bristle.

Facilities
Facilities should take account of cultural needs. For example, the waiting area should be appropriate for accompanying people such as children or families, and if divided discretely can permit women to sit alone if need be. Toilet facilities should permit perineal washing for those people, such as Muslims, who prefer this. This could be a simple ancillary (bidet) shower, a bidet, or one of the more sophisticated water closets that have perineal washing facility. Separate soap and towels should be provided for use on the upper and lower parts of the body; disposable items should be provided.

Relevant Websites

http://aad.english.ucsb.edu/pages/culture.html (The AAD Project bibliography of culture and affirmative action)

http://www.bbc.co.uk/religion/religions (BBC guide to religion and ethics) http://www.diversityrx.org/HTML/MOCPT2.htm [L-E-A-R-N (Listen, explain, acknowledge, recommend, negotiate) model of cross cultural encounter guidelines for health practitioners]

Religions and Faiths

Aim

This section presents outlines of various religions and faiths that may be encountered, giving details of holidays, holy days and festivals, together with generalised information on dietary and other habits and restrictions, health and healing traditions and oral healthcare issues.

Outcome

This section should come to be viewed as a source of reference to enhance culturally sensitive healthcare through knowledge and understanding of different religions.

Overview

Patients' views, reactions to illness, health needs and expectations of treatment vary widely and are influenced by many factors, of which religious beliefs may be but one.

Religious convictions and beliefs may govern a patient's life or, at the other extreme, have limited, if any, influence on their views, needs and wishes. Furthermore, a patient's attitude towards their religion, its beliefs and practices may change with time, or as a consequence of life events, including, for example, the diagnosis of certain illnesses and bereavement.

Healthcare providers (HCPs) must be sensitive to such issues to best relate to patients and to avoid possible criticisms of insensitivity, let alone run the risk of giving offence.

Certain religious beliefs and practices may be viewed as barriers to best possible clinical outcomes and thereby present the HCP with ethical problems. Such situations are best managed by carefully listening to the individual patient's needs, wishes and concerns, and through discussions between patient and HCPs as to how best to address possible conflicts and dilemmas.

The HCP must never make assumptions based on generalisations. Health and health beliefs and practices are discussed here from a traditional perspective, understanding that individuals may subscribe to all, some or even none of them.

Patients must be treated as individuals, never stereotyped. It is crucial to remember that there is considerable variation in every religious group. If in doubt, enquire as to the specific needs and wishes of the individual patient and take time to discuss and describe the proposed treatment. Good communications are central to effective culturally sensitive care.

The healthcare professional must never discriminate against a patient for whatever reason, including religious beliefs. Differences in religious beliefs between patient and HCP must be set aside, with the interests of the patient being put first and foremost.

Religions and Faiths

Religion is a difference that tends to matter. Religions and faiths have a variable effect on human behaviour, but often have more influence than cultural, ethnic or other factors.

There is a multitude of religions and faiths in the world. Discussion here is limited to the majority religions and faiths. There are more than two hundred other different religious groups and movements: detail can be found at http://religiousmovements.lib.virginia.edu/

Non-Believers

In practical terms, non-believers in a god often follow the same moral code as religious people, but arrive at decisions of what is good or bad without help or reference to God or scriptures.

Non-believers usually encourage the celebration of the major events in life, including namings, weddings and funerals, giving meaning and significance to such occasions without any religious content.

Agnosticism
Agnostics are people who have doubts about the existence of God.

Atheism

Atheism is not a belief; rather it is both the absence of belief in God and a denial of the existence of God. The various types of atheism include:

- *Buddhism* – a way of living based on the teachings of Siddartha Gautama
- *Christian Non-realism* – a form of Christianity without an external God
- *Humanism* – a philosophy that teaches that it is immoral not to act to stop wars, crimes and brutality
- *Humanistic Judaism* – a form of Judaism without God
- *Post-modernism* – a view of religion without God, and without any absolute values
- *Rationalism* – an approach to life based on reason and evidence
- *Secularism* – emphasises that no-one should be disadvantaged for not having a religious faith
- *Unitarianism or Universalism* – a form of individual belief, most of whose members adopt a non-realist position and focus on humankind as the source of religious authority

Non–Believers and Healthcare

In general, non-believers have few if any dietary restrictions, habits, health and healing traditions or health and illness practices that influence the delivery of oral healthcare provision. Non-believers rarely object to others, including HCPs, having religious beliefs, assuming such beliefs do not influence treatment planning and the subsequent provision of care.

Religions (Faiths)

There are numerous beliefs (religions or faiths) in the world and, with increasing multiculturalism, numerous faiths exist in most countries (Fig 2-1). Indigenous faiths are also practised, especially in many developing countries.

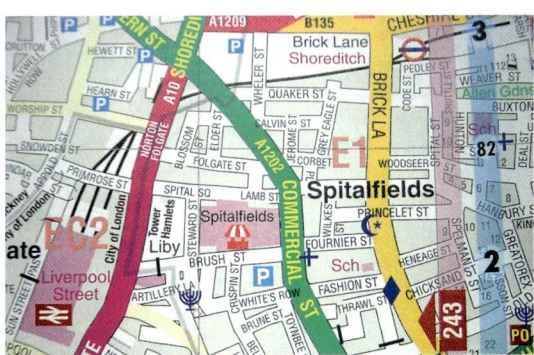

Fig 2-1 London map showing proximity of synagogues, mosque and churches.

59

The most common religions in developed countries include, in descending order of frequency worldwide:
• Christianity
• Islam
• Hinduism
• Sikhism
• Judaism
• Buddhism
• Jainism

This section discusses these and some other less common religions, in particular as to how they do, or do not affect healthcare (Table 2-1).

The most important periods recognised in most religions and faiths are birth, reaching maturity, marriage and death. Most religions also have holy days, at which times elective healthcare is best avoided.

African Religions

Background
African religions refer mainly to religions that have their origins in sub-Saharan Africa. They are practised largely in Africa, and by some people of African heritage living elsewhere, especially in Haiti and some other parts of the Caribbean. They may be practised alone, but are often practised along with Christianity or other traditions. They may be practised overtly or covertly.

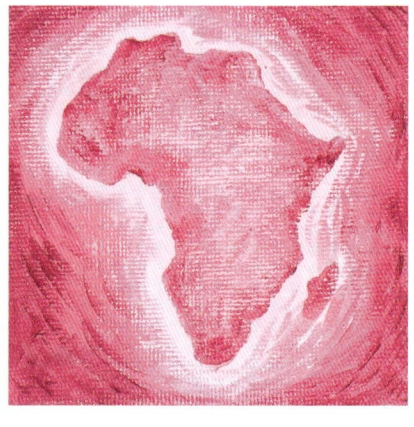

African religions have derived mainly from West Africa and the culture of the Yoruba – a number of semi-independent peoples loosely linked by geography, language, history and religion. These Yoruba faiths have given origin to other religions in the Americas and elsewhere where African- based cultures exist, and include:
• Ifaism – the major faith is usually referred to as Yoruba and honours several deities.
• Voodou (also known as Vodun, Voodoo (pejorative), Vodou and Vodoun) – has been influenced by Roman Catholic traditions as well as by the Spiritism movement under the banner of Kardecism. Popular mis-

Table 2-1 **The bases of the main religions**

Religion	Basis
Bahá'í	A young religion based on Islam
Buddhism	A type of atheism and way of living based on teachings of Siddartha Gautama
Christianity	A group of faiths based on the teaching of Jesus Christ
Hinduism	A group of faiths rooted in religious ideas of India
Islam	A religion based on the teaching of prophet Muhammad
Jainism	An ancient philosophy and ethical teaching originating in India
Judaism	A religion based around the Jewish people's covenant relationship with God
Mormonism	The Church of Jesus Christ of Latter-day Saints
Paganism	Contemporary religions usually based on reverence for nature
Rastafarianism	A religion based on the teaching of Marcus Garvey
Shinto	A religion with its origins in Japan based on no known founder or single sacred scripture
Sikhism	A religion based on the teaching of Guru Nanak
Unitarianism	An open-minded and individualistic approach to religion
Zoroastrianism	An Iranian-based religion stemming from the teaching of prophet Zoroaster

conceptions about voodou have created somewhat of a negative stereotype. It is a religion based on family spirits who generally help and protect. Although lacking a fixed theology and an organized hierarchy, voodou is a religion with its own rituals, ceremonies, and altars that practitioners do not find to be at odds with Roman Catholicism. For example, pictures of Catholic saints are painted on the walls of temples to represent the voodou spirits; at funerals, it is not uncommon that voodou ceremonies and rituals are performed for family members first, followed by a more public traditional Roman Catholic ceremony presided over by a priest. Voodou is derived from a synthesis of African religious beliefs. These spirits, or loas, are inherited or bought by families and can be called upon for help; they can be paid to bring good fortune and protect, or to attack enemies. Payment is usually in the form of food, drink or other gifts offered during rituals.
- Santeria - evolved mainly in Cuba and is now found throughout the Americas. Except, perhaps, for the ritual sacrifice of animals, in particular chickens, it differs little from other Ifa-derived religions.

Other African religions have derived from the culture of Bantu and others in the Congo, Zaire and Angola. They have given origin to other religions in the Americas (mainly Brazil and Cuba) and elsewhere that African-based cultures exist. They include:
- Kongo
- Palo Monte
- Palo Mayombe
- Xango (Shango)
- Quimbanda
- Umbanda.

Beliefs
There is a belief in various spirits believed to play a part in health and other aspects of life.

Main Religious Days
African religions have many, different religious days, the main ones being:
- Cassé Gâteau – January
- Tirer Gâteau (Les rois) - January
- Norriture Rituelle des sources têt d' l'eau – February
- Loco Davi (manger du bois rituel) – March
- Legba Zaou – March

- Dan Wè Zo, alias St Louis Cleimeille – April
- Cassé Canari ou Wèt mô nan d'lo – April
- Mangé les Morts – April
- Mangers pour divers loas – May
- Manger pour Gran'n Aloumandia – May
- Simbi Blanc – May
- St. Jean's Day – June
- Papa Ogou (St Jacques le Majeur) – July
- Gran'Délai et Gran'Aloumandia (Sainte Anne) – July
- Maitresse Silverine – July
- Table Communion pour Dan Wezo, Roi de France – August
- Agou – August
- Roi Wangol, Mousindi – September
- Manman Aloumandia – September
- Maitresse Délai – September
- Chanté – messes – October
- All Saint's Day – November
- All Soul's Day – November
- Mangé Yam (Fête de la moisson) – November
- Ganga – Bois – December
- Agoué - Arroyo (Mangé la mer) – December
- Bain de Noêl (Frotté feuilles) or Fête des Membres - December

In general, it is best to avoid treatment on these days. If this is not possible, the patient should be asked to give details of things to be avoided.

Dietary and other Habits and Restrictions
African meals tend to include potatoes, rice, corn or yams, with green vegetables and meat. Some Africans prefer 'bush meat' (e.g. monkey meat). Traditionally, the largest meal is on Sundays.

Main Languages
There is no predominant language.

Modesty
Depends on religion.

Attitudes to Healthcare Professionals
The patient may expect the HCP to have all the answers and make all the decisions, and may be reluctant to openly disagree with HCPs.

Health and Healing Traditions

It is difficult to separate African religions from African medicine: many 'traditional healers' are also religious leaders and vice versa.

Traditional healers use both scientific and subjective knowledge. Traditional medicines are obtained mainly from plants (as of course, are many scientific medicines). The major sources of non-scientific or subjective knowledge are the various spirits, often ancestral, believed to play a part in health.

In providing treatment, efforts should be made to avoid negating positive outcomes of such social and psychological methods of treatment, possibly through rejection of such approaches. Africans will sometimes consult both types of healers concurrently, with traditional healers being thought of as addressing the 'ultimate' (i.e. spiritual) causes of the affliction.

Oral Healthcare Issues

An underlying suspicion of ways in which drugs affect the body and bodily functions may be addressed by an explanation of the mechanisms and effects of any intended drugs. Otherwise, there is typically acceptance of routine dental care. Restrictions on healthcare provision vary with the religion and the religious conviction. In general, there are restrictions on receipt of blood products. There may be a reluctance to agree to surgery.

Relevant Websites

http://www.ligali.org (Ligali, the African British Equality Authority home page.)

http://www.wcc-coe.org/wcc/what/interreligious/cd33-02.html (World Council of Churches Christianity, African religion and African medicine.)

http://members.aol.com/porchfour/religion/african.htm (Information on African religions and their derivatives.)

Bahá'í Faith

Background

Bahá'í is one of the newest world religions. Founded by Bahá'u'lláh, a 19th-century Iranian exile, it emerged from Islam. It is perhaps unique in that it unreservedly accepts the validity of other faiths.

Beliefs
Bahá'ís believe that all people are integral parts of one divine plan. They encourage world peace by teaching tolerance and promoting:

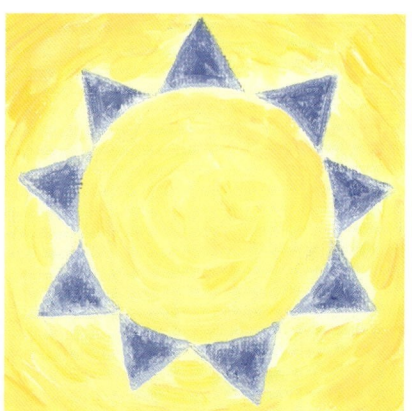

- abandonment of all forms of prejudice
- assurance to women of full equality of opportunity with men
- recognition of the unity and relativity of religious truth
- elimination of extremes of poverty and wealth
- realization of universal education
- responsibility of each person to independently search for truth
- establishment of a global commonwealth of nations
- recognition that true religion is in harmony with reason and the pursuit of scientific knowledge.

Worship
Bahá'ís have no ordained clergy or fixed services of worship. They say an obligatory prayer daily, facing Bahji – near Akka in Israel, and read their holy scriptures in the morning and evening.

Holy Days and Festivals
The main holidays and festivals when treatment should, if possible, be avoided, include:
- Fast of Nineteen Days – March
- Feast of Naw-Ruz (New Year) – March
- First day of Ridvan (Declaration of Bahaullah) – April
- Ninth day of Ridvan – April
- Twelfth day of Ridvan – May
- Birth of Abdul-Baha – May
- Declaration of the Bab – May
- Ascension of Bahaullah – May
- Martyrdom of the Bab – July
- Birth of the Bab – October
- Birth of Bahaullah – November
- Day of the Covenant – November
- Ascension of Abdul-Baha - November

- The holy days that require Bahá'ís to refrain from work are the three special days of Ridvan (1st, 9th, 12th).

Dietary and other Habits and Restrictions
- Bahá'ís do not drink alcohol or take habit-forming drugs, and tend to avoid eating pork. Smoking is discouraged.

Main Languages
There is no predominant language.

Ideas of Modesty
Bahá'ís rarely object to opposite-gender HCPs.

Attitudes to Healthcare Professionals
Bahá'ís are usually positive towards HCPs.

Health and Healing traditions
The Bahá'í faith has many health and healing traditions and remedies but these rarely preclude or counteract drugs and procedures which may be employed in western oral healthcare provision. Attempts to discredit traditional medicines and remedies may be viewed with suspicion.

Bahá'ís are forbidden to take drugs other than for medical reasons. When prescribing drugs, care may need to be taken to reassure patients that the effects of the drugs are not intended to counteract the effects of traditional medicines. They can accept or donate blood and organs.

Oral Healthcare Issues
Routine dental care should pose no problem, provided alcohol and pork-containing products are avoided, but some members of the faith may decline the administration of blood products. Bahá'ísm accepts healthcare measures and procedures that help promote the main tennets of the faith.

Relevant Website
http://www.bahai.org/ (The International Website of the Bahá'í Faith)

Buddhism

Background
Buddhism is a monastic atheistic system founded in India by Siddhartha Gautama (the Buddha), now represented by many groups, especially numerous

in Asia. These groups profess varying forms of the doctrine and venerate Buddha. About 550 million Buddhists now live in Asia, from Sri Lanka and Thailand in the south, through South-East Asia to Tibet, China, Japan, Korea, Russia and Mongolia in the north.

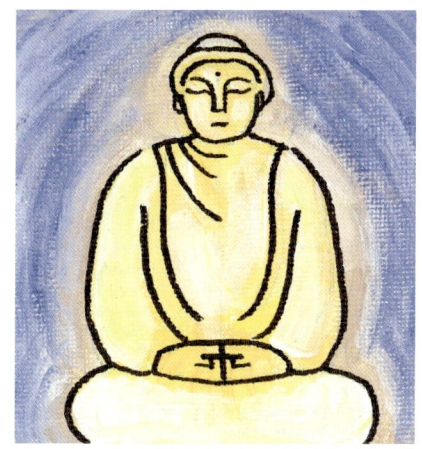

Buddhism is divided into the Theravada or Hinayana, found mainly in Sri Lanka and south east Asia, and the Mahayana found in China, Mongolia, Korea, and Japan. A third school, the Vajrayana, has a long tradition in Tibet and Japan.

Beliefs

Buddhism sees life as a process of birth, ageing, illness and death in which people seek enlightenment. It has tended to merge into the everyday life of the countries where it has taken root and is characterised by a spirit of gentleness, forgiveness of injuries, cultivation of benevolence towards people of all classes, avoidance of anger and violence, patience under insult, and the return of good for evil. Buddhists believe that radiating loving kindness to all living beings is a practice that benefits oneself and all others.

The Buddha's teaching are based on The Four Noble Truths and The Eightfold Path, which lead Buddhists towards the path of Enlightenment (the right understanding, thought, speech, action, livelihood, effort, mindfulness and concentration).

Venerating the Buddha and exchanging gifts are fundamental customs. Many Buddhists wear a string or chain around the neck with an amulet containing a Buddhist transcript for protection.

Worship

Instead of worship of a creator or God, Buddhism teaches that the individual must find in oneself the solution to true happiness by developing the qualities of awareness, kindness and wisdom. Buddhists practise meditation, to develop more positive states of mind characterised by calmness, concentration, awareness and emotions such as friendliness.

Holy Days and Festivals

All Buddhist religious festivals follow the lunar calendar, the main ones being celebrated on full-moon days. The most important include:

- Wesak - the most important festival, celebrates the birth, enlightenment and death of the Buddha. It is celebrated on the full moon in May.
- Dharma Day - marks the beginning of the Buddha's teaching.
- Sangha Day - celebrates the Buddhist spiritual community
- Parinirvana Day - a Mahayana festival marking the death of the Buddha.
- Losar - most important holiday in Tibet, celebrating the Tibetan New Year.
- Fasting may occur on some of these days, especially on new moon and full moon days, and Wesak. Nevertheless, there is a huge diversity in range of festivals and ceremonies.

Dietary and Other Habits and Restrictions

No intoxicants or alcohol are permitted. Many Buddhists are vegetarians, in accordance with the belief that no living creature should be harmed, but in the Theravada tradition meat is an accepted part of the diet.

Ideas of Modesty

There are no special issues.

Attitudes to Healthcare Professionals

These are generally positive.

Health and Healing Traditions

Buddhism accepts physical ailments as an inevitable part of life. Buddhists tend to accept fate and suffering with stoicism, behavioural reserve and suppression of negative thoughts and complaints.

Traditional medicines are popular. Although western healthcare is often the main mode of treatment used, alternative forms of therapy tend also to be sought, especially where western methods fail.

Buddhists do not like any medication. Those who follow vegan or vegetarian diets may object to the use of animal products to meet the needs of humans. Blood transfusions are accepted. Organ transplantation is a complex issue.

Oral Healthcare Issues

The Buddhist tendency to accept fate and suffering may discourage dental attendance. Stoicism may be displayed through reluctance to accept pain relief. Where indicated, the need and indications for pain relief should be carefully explained to the patient. Specific consent should be sought to administer local analgesia. When treatment is provided, the use of blood, alcohol and animal products should be avoided.

Relevant Website
http://www.thebuddhistsociety.org/ (General website about Buddhism and the Buddhist Society of the UK.)

Christianity

Background
Founded two thousand years ago in the Middle East, when Jesus Christ and his followers began their mission within the context of Judaism. Christianity appeared as a separate religion with its own scriptures, laws, and institutional and ritual forms after attracting large numbers of adherents from the many non-Semitic races in the Mediterranean world.

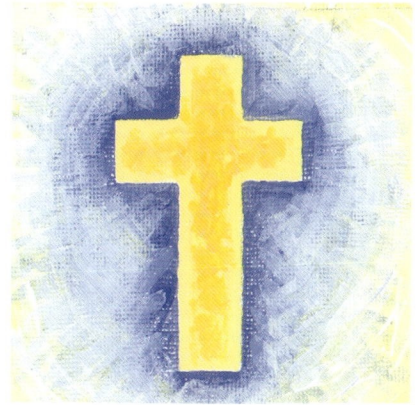

Christianity is a major world religion, found in most countries, in particular the Americas, Europe, Commonwealth of Independent States (CIS), Central and Southern Africa, the Far East and Australasia (Figs 2-2 and 2-3). Christianity divided first between Catholic in the West and Orthodox in the East; later between Roman Catholic and Protestantism, when there was disruption into a multitude of denominations. The main Christian churches are shown in Table 2-2.

Beliefs
A Christian is one who professes belief in Jesus as Christ or Messiah, or follows a religion based on the life and teachings of Jesus. Christians believe that the son of God was Jesus Christ, a Jew who lived during the Roman occupation of Israel, and whose creed was to love God and to love one's neighbour as oneself. Jesus was crucified, and Christians believe he was resurrected on the third day after his death, and after 40 days ascended into heaven. All Christians believe in God and the divinity of Christ, but nevertheless there are significant differences between different groups of Christians.

69

Table 2-2 **Main Christian churches**

Churches	Main examples
Anglicans	Church of England
	Scottish Episcopal Church
	Church of Ireland
	Church in Wales
Eastern orthodox	Coptic orthodox Church
	Ethiopian orthodox Church
	Greek orthodox Church
	Russian orthodox Church
	Serbian orthodox Church
	Syrian orthodox Church
Protestant (Free and non-conformists)	Adventist Church
	Baptist Church
	Church of Christ
	Church of Scotland
	Congregational Church
	Elim Church
	God of Prophecy Church
	Lutheran Church
	Methodist Church
	Moravian Church
	New Testament Church
	Pentacostal Church
	Plymouth Brethren
	Presbyterian Church
	Quaker Church (Society of Friends)
	Salvation Army
	Unitarian Church
	United Reformed Church
Roman Catholic	

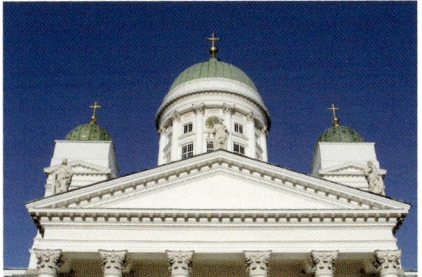

Fig 2-2 Christian church in Scandinavia.

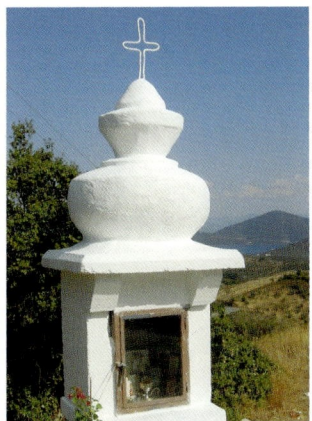

Fig 2-3 Christian icon in the Balkans.

Many Christians use the New Testament as their holy book; others also use the Old Testament. Christening (baptism) is a ceremony at the start of an individual's relationship with God, and takes place at a range of ages.

Culture
The cross of Christ's crucifixion is the main Christian symbol. In addition, the ancient Christians' symbol was the sign of the fish. In general, Christianity rarely prescribes precise details of personal life such as diet or dress, but marriage and family life are important, with views varying on divorce, homosexuality, contraception, abortion etc.

Christians usually have a personal name or two, followed by a shared family name. Women typically take their husband's family name on marriage, and children take their father's family name.

Holy Days and Festivals
Sunday is generally regarded as a day of rest and those who support churches attend them. The main holy days include:
• Advent (Approach) (December); four week preparation to commemorate the coming of God to earth as Christ
• Christmas and Epiphany (Manifestation) (December); the birth of Jesus Christ
• Lent (February / March); six-week preparation for death and resurrection of Christ. The 1st Day of Lent is The Great Feast (Orthodox)
• Holy week and Easter (March /April/ May)

Table 2-3 **Oral healthcare issues in Christian groups**

Christian groups	Tea & coffee	Alcohol	Tobacco	Restricted items Blood and blood products	Hypnotism	Animal products
Adventists	✓	✓	✓	✓	✓	✓ (some)
Christian Scientists	✓ (some)	✓	✓	✓		✓ (some)
Jehovah's Witnesses			✓	✓		✓ (some)
Mormons	✓	✓	✓			

✓ = restricted

- Palm Sunday, Maundy Thursday and Good Friday recall the last days of Christ's life on earth before crucifixion.
- Easter Sunday recalls Christ's resurrection from the dead.
- Ascension Day recalls Christ's ascension into heaven
- Whit Sunday recalls Pentecost and the coming of the Holy Spirit
- Trinity Sunday commemorates the Trinity; Father, Son and Holy Ghost.

Dietary and Other Habits and Restrictions
There are no universal requirements, but some Christians choose to eat fish rather than meat on Fridays, especially in Lent. The 40 days of Lent (between Ash Wednesday and Easter) have traditionally been a period of abstinence; but observance has diminished greatly in recent years. Christianity did not develop elaborate dietary rules and customs, and any dietary restrictions are normally a matter of personal choice or related to medical conditions.

Main Languages
Various.

Ideas of Modesty
There are no special issues.

Attitudes to Healthcare Professionals
These are generally positive.

Health and Healing Traditions
Most Christians accept healthcare willingly.

Oral Healthcare Issues
Acceptance of dental care is high, although attitudes to oral health and dental attendance are variable, but mainly for cultural and social reasons.

The Christian groups whose beliefs may impact on oral healthcare include the Adventists, Christian Scientists, Jehovah's witnesses and Mormons (Table 2-3, and below).

Adventism

Background
Adventism, which arose from the works of William Miller in 1831, is a group of six predominantly American Protestant sects that include:
- Evangelical Adventists (the original group)

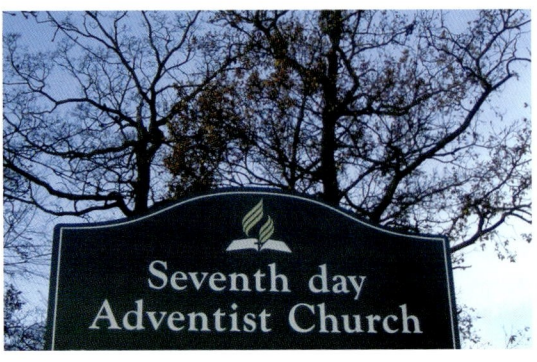

Fig 2-4 The main Adventist church.

- Seventh Day Adventists (Fig 2-4)
- The Church of God
- Advent Christians
- Life and Advent Union
- Age-to-come Adventists
- Beliefs
- The common belief of Adventism is in the Bible and the imminent return of Christ.

Holy Days and Festivals
Sabbath is Saturday, so treatment should be avoided on Friday evening and Saturday until sunset.

Dietary and Other Habits and Restrictions
Adventists take no alcohol, coffee or tea; they tend to be vegetarian, some are vegan, and few eat pork or shellfish. Narcotics, tobacco and other stimulants are banned.

Health and Healing Traditions
Adventists believe that the body must be kept healthy. Their diet and lifestyle appear to confer significant longevity. Some patients, particularly those who follow vegan or vegetarian diets, may object to the use of animals to meet the needs of humans.

Oral Healthcare Issues
Hypnotism is banned, but dental care is otherwise freely accepted. Products containing alcohol or animal derivatives should be avoided.

Christian Scientists

Dietary and Other Habits and Restrictions
Christian Scientists avoid alcohol and tobacco, and some avoid tea and coffee.

Health and Healing Traditions
Christian Scientists believe that there is no disease that is beyond the power of God to heal, and thus they believe in spiritual healing. They do not like tests, medicines or drugs, blood transfusions, surgery, or organ transplants – or to prolong life. Vaccines are accepted only as much as to keep within the law.

Oral Healthcare Issues
Dental care is typically well accepted and, with the above possible constraints, no difficulties should be encountered in the provision of routine care. Products containing alcohol are best avoided.

Jehovah's Witnesses

Jehovah's witnesses regard Jesus Christ as son of God, but they do not recognise the traditional holy days of other Christian groups, such as Sundays, Christmas and Easter. Bible study is important to them, and they accept both Old and New Testaments. Jehovah's witnesses shun the use of the cross.

Beliefs
Jehovah's witnesses have a strong belief that an individual must not sustain his or her life with another creature's blood.

Worship
Jehovah's witnesses worship in Kingdom Halls.

Holy Days and Festivals
Jehovah witnesses have an annual ceremony, the Memorial.

Dietary and Other Habits and Restrictions
Jehovah's witnesses believe it wrong to eat blood, so products such as black pudding are not eaten. When meat is eaten it must be washed clean of all blood and well cooked. Some are vegetarian. Jehovah's witnesses use no tobacco and little alcohol.

Health and Healing Traditions
The prohibition against blood includes transfusions of:
- whole blood
- red cells
- white cells
- platelets
- plasma.

However, albumin, coagulation factors, immunoglobulins, autotransfusion, haemodialysis and extracorporeal bypass, and vaccination, provided no other person's blood is used, are exempt. Erythropoietin has been used to circumvent the problem. Because of their belief against blood transfusion, Jehovah Witnesses are often (wrongly) presumed to be opposed to tissue and organ donation, but this merely means that all blood must be removed from the organs and tissues before being transplanted.

If surgery is planned and there is any possibility of serious haemorrhage, the matter should be discussed and arrangements agreed with the patient preoperatively. Most Jehovah's witnesses carry a card (Advance Medical Directive/Release) directing against blood transfusion and releasing HCPs from responsibilities in this regard.

Jehovah's Witness Hospital Liaison Committees or the local Watchtower Society can often help with questions about life-prolonging measures.

Oral Healthcare Issues
Dental care is typically well accepted, and no difficulties should be encountered in the provision of routine care. Some patients, in particular those who follow vegan or vegetarian diets, may object to the use of animals to meet the needs of humans, so animal-free products are best used.

Mormonism (Church of Jesus Christ of Latter-day Saints)
Background
Mormonism was founded by Joseph Smith, the son of a farmer in the USA. Smith, in order to satisfy himself as to which Methodist sect he should join, sought Divine guidance. He claimed to have received the answer in a visitation from two glorious beings, who told him not to connect himself to any sect, but to bide the coming of the Church of Christ. This he eventually founded in Salt Lake City, Utah.

Beliefs
Old and New Testaments together with the book of Mormonism are the holy scriptures. Family unity is important. Mormons claim the privilege of worshipping God according to the dictates of their conscience, and worshiping how, where, or what they may. Mormons believe in being honest, true, chaste, benevolent and virtuous and in doing good to all men. The Church opposes pornography and immorality, and teaches sexual purity before marriage and faithfulness during marriage. Polygamy was a founding principle of the creed and, although not enforced by the laws of the Mormon hierarchy, was previously preached by the elders and practised by many.

Worship
There are no paid ministers and the members serve a 'calling' from time to time.

Dietary and Other Habits and Restrictions
There is a code termed 'Word of Wisdom', which warns against use of stimulants. Thus Mormons avoid alcohol, tobacco, tea, coffee, caffeine in soft drinks and habit-forming drugs. Mormons fast once a month.

Health and Healing Traditions
Views about herbal medicine are varied. Mormons may wear a 'garment' as underclothing, which should not be removed without consent. The church encourages blood donation, but the question of organ transplantation (donation or receipt) is left to the individual.

Oral Healthcare Issues
Little, if any, difficulties may be anticipated in the provision of routine dental care to Mormons. Alcohol-containing products should be avoided, as should the prescription of alcohol-containing mouthwashes (see Table 1-8).

Pentacostalism

Most Pentacostalists are of Caribbean origin, and believe in, and practise, strong moral codes of behaviour. Most are modest and expect privacy.

Holy Days and Festivals
Sunday is the day for congregational worship. Easter is the main religious festival.

Dietary Restrictions and Habits
Fasting is commonplace amongst Pentacostalists, but the timing is variable.

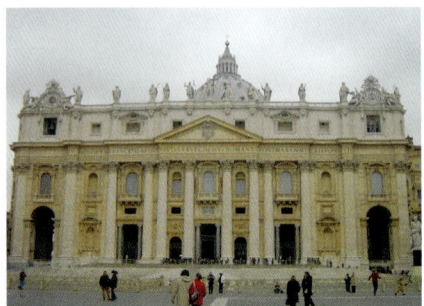

Fig 2-5 St Peters (Rome), the main Roman Catholic church.

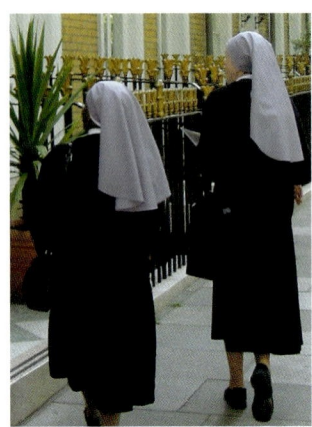

Fig 2-6 Nuns.

Catholicism (Roman Catholicism)

Background
The Church of Rome (Roman Catholicism) split with Orthodox Christians in 1054 over questions of doctrine and the absolute authority and behaviour of the Pope. Catholicism is centred on the City of Rome (Fig 2-5 and Fig 2-6). There are more than a billion Catholics worldwide, with particular concentrations in southern Europe, Central and South America, the United States and the Philippines.

Beliefs
Catholics share with other Christians a belief in the divinity of Jesus Christ, but organisation and teachings differ.

Holy Days and Festivals
Sunday mass is the main religious service; confession is a sacrament at which people confess their sins to a priest and are given absolution (forgiveness) on the understanding these sins are not to be repeated. Other religious days are as for most other Christians.

Dietary and Other Habits and Restrictions
Catholics may, on Fridays, eat fish rather than meat. Most fast, or at least abstain from meat and alcohol, on Ash Wednesday and Good Friday.

Health and Healing Traditions
There is a strong belief in the ability of prayer to help healing.

78

Oral Healthcare Issues
No special precautions or arrangements need apply in the provision of dental care to Catholics.

Relevant Websites
http://www.bbc.co.uk/religion/religions/christianity/index.shtml (BBC guide to religion and ethics Christianity section)

http://home.christianity.com/(General site about Christianity, with a section on other religions)

http://dmoz.org/Society/Religion_and_Spirituality/Christianity/ (Many thousands of links to websites about Christianity)

Confucianism

Background
Confucius (K'ung Fu-tzu), a Chinese philosopher from about 2500 years ago, created Confucianism, based on ancient Chinese traditions. It is practised mainly by peoples from east Asia, especially China and surrounding areas. Elements of Confucianism also survive in Taiwan, Hong Kong and Macao.

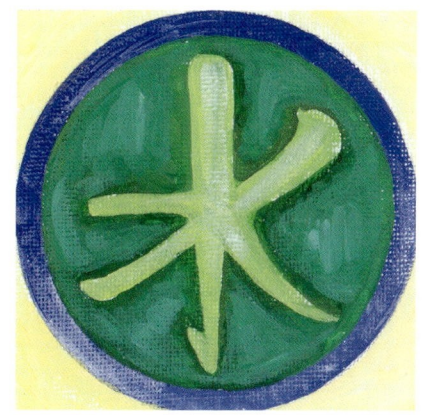

Beliefs
Confucianism is more of an ethical system rather than a religion, which emphasises law and respect for authority and rules as central to life. Confucianism concentrates on interpersonal rules and the proper way to conduct social interactions, reminding people to practise moderation, avoid excess, understand that they are destined to fulfill a mission on earth and need to allow fate (ming) to guide their lives. The key teachings are:
• reciprocity (pao; one should treat others as one wants to be treated)
• loyalty (chung).

These teachings have led to a respect for authority and a demand for filial piety. This manifests itself in young people respecting and obeying the wishes of their parents and other elders, with unquestioning allegiance and subordination to one's elders and authority figures.

Holy Days and Festivals
The birth of Confucius is usually celebrated in September.

Main languages
See Chinese

Ideas of Modesty
See Chinese

Attitudes to Healthcare Professionals
See Chinese

Health and Healing Traditions
See Chinese

Oral Healthcare Issues
In general, attitudes towards western healthcare are similar to those found amongst the Chinese (see Chinese). Traditional Chinese medicine may be preferred or used in conjunction with western medicine. Some followers of Confucianism believe in spiritual healing. Oral healthcare may be a relatively low priority for Confucians.

Falun Dafa and Falun Gong

Background
Falun Gong consists of a set of five exercises that promote one's cultivation; three of the exercises involve movements and manoeuvres while the other two require remaining still for extended periods of time. Falun Dafa is a movement with no leader, and there is no form of worship or rituals, and it is not involved with politics. Nevertheless, it is persecuted in some places (Fig 2-7).

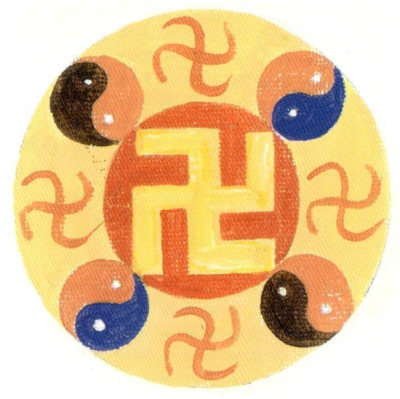

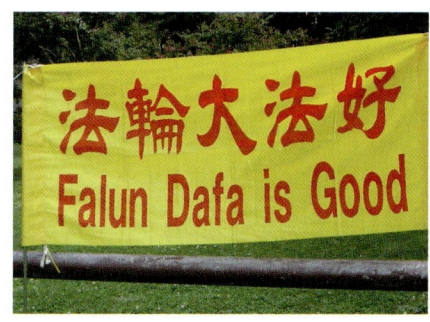

Fig 2-7 Falun Dafa poster.

Beliefs
The Falun movement only accepts heterosexual behaviour.

Main languages
See Chinese

Ideas of Modesty
See Chinese

Attitudes to Healthcare Professionals
See Chinese

Health and Healing Traditions
Falun followers believe that clinical tests and examinations cannot detect the fundamental cause of an illness. Rather they believe that karma is the cause of illness and that the body's vital energy, Qi, can be focused to improve one's health and sense of well-being and can also be used to heal diseases.

Oral Healthcare Issues
Acceptance of western healthcare, including dental healthcare, may be limited, in particular when illness takes the form of, for example, infection. Treatments which followers believe to reduce Qi should be avoided.

Relevant Website
http://www.religioustolerance.org/falungong.htm (Information about Falun Gong and Falun Dafa in China and elsewhere. Also some information about Buddhism and Taoism.)

Hinduism

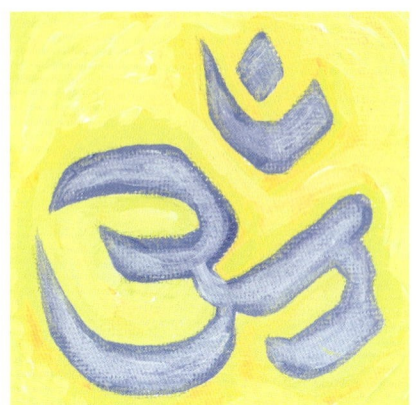

Background

Hinduism is the main Indian religion, the third largest world religion after Christianity and Islam, with almost one billion followers. Nevertheless, Hinduism is unique in being a national, rather than a world religion. The roots of Hinduism lie in the Indus (Sindhu) valley in Northern India (Hindustan) over 8500 years ago. Hinduism is most dominant in Assam, Bengal, Berrar, Chennai, Mumbai, Agra, Oudh and the Central Provinces.

Beliefs

Hinduism may be considered a 'way of life' rather than an organised religion. It includes a wide range of beliefs and practices, focussed on the equality of all humans, regardless of caste, colour and creed, and respect and reverence for womanhood. Hindus aim to live in a way that will cause each of their lives to be better than the life before. Their five guiding principles are:
• truth
• correct conduct
• peace
• righteousness
• non–violence (ahinsa).

Care and concern for all beings is fundamental: major duties include obedience to parents and care and respect for elders. The Hindu sign – the Aum – represents the three stages of life: birth, life and death, while the swastika is for good luck and prosperity. Hindu sects include Advaitaism, Swaminarayanism and Vedanta.

Worship

Hindus believe that there is one supreme God called Brahma who is present in all things and gives all living things life. There are many aspects of Brahma, including gods such as Mahadeva, Parvati, Shakti, Shiva and Vishnu. Hindus also have a strong belief in astrology and believe in Dharma (destiny in life) and Karma - the natural law of reward or punishment for thoughts and deeds.

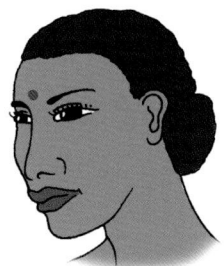

Fig 2-8 Kukum – denoting a married woman.

Many Hindus pray (Pujah) at least three times daily, on waking, at noon and at sunset, and also often before meals. They usually wash before prayers. Many Hindus also meet for festivals at temples or mandirs, but there are no regular church meetings.

Culture
Family values are central and many Hindus live in an extended family, in which every member has a role, often determined by age and gender. Elders help guide younger family members in choices regarding career, marriage and finances. Children can look forward to continual family support but, in return, are expected to respect family ties and wishes and to support parents in their advancing years. Hindus hold family progress, unity and support in high regard.

A large number of marriages are arranged by parents. A chain of gold and black glass beads (the 'mangalsutra' or 'thali') is given by the husband to his wife at the time of their wedding. A married Hindu woman can be recognised by her mangalsutra, which is worn throughout married life – like a ring in Christian marriages. A married Hindu woman is also supposed to have a vermilion mark, 'the kukum', on her forehead (Fig 2-8), and to wear bangles. It is considered very inauspicious for a married woman to be seen without these. If widowed, however, the mangalsutra, vermilion mark and bangles are removed. Men may wear a tattoo or necklace (Figs 2-9 and 2-10). Divorce is strongly disapproved of.

Traditionally, Hindu men support their families. Many women also contribute to the family's income but, even if they have careers, women are largely responsible for maintaining the household and caring for children and aged relatives.

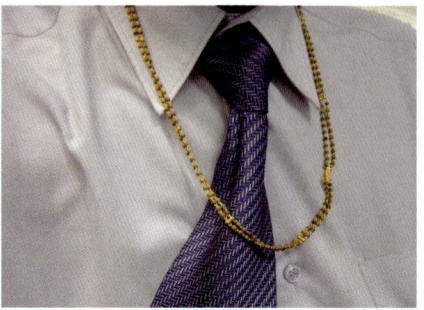
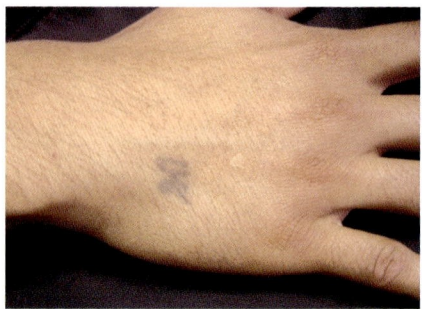

Fig 2-9 Hindu necklace. **Fig 2-10** Hindu tattoo.

Most Hindus use a personal name (e.g. Vyomesh), a complementary name (e.g. for men, Bhai, Chand, Das, Dev, Kant, Kumar, Lal, Nat, Pal; for women, Behn, Devi, Gowri, Kumari, Lakshmi, Rani) and a family name (e.g. Patel).

Hindu women traditionally wear a sari over a blouse and underskirt. Men tend to wear conventional Western clothing, with traditional clothing reserved for family events and special occasions. Many young Indians have adopted Western clothing styles. Traditionally, North Indian men wear a kameez (loose shirt) and pyjamas (trousers), while a dhoti (cloth around waist drawn between legs) or lungi (cloth around waist) are favored by South Indian men. Many Hindus wear a 'protective' sacred thread on the right wrist or torso – which should not be removed. Swaminarayans wear a Kanthi (necklace) of sandalwood, which should not be removed.

The Hindu social caste system, which is less used nowadays, groups people as shown in Table 2-4.

Holy Days and Festivals
Hindu festivals are largely linked with the movements of the sun and moon and seasonal changes. The important festivals are;
• Diwali (Deepawali) – the main festival, a festival of lights celebrating the New Year between late October and mid-November, and lasting five days.
• Dasara – ten days of celebration of the triumph of good over evil in honour of Durga or Kali, held between late September and mid-October.
• Holi – the spring festival in March celebrating creation and renewal.

Table 2-4 **Hindu caste system**

Caste	Includes
Brahmins	Priests
Kshatriyas	Warriors
Vaishyas	Merchants
Sudras	Labourers

Pilgrimage is also an important aspect of Hinduism, particularly to the Ganges and other rivers. Different Hindus hold different festivals and prioritise them differently as well. It is always best to therefore ask the individual what specific holy days he/she observes.

Dietary and Other Habits and Restrictions
Hindus believe they should eat nothing that involves violence to any living thing. This often leads to vegetarianism. Hindus will not eat beef; some will not eat eggs; others will not eat dairy produce. Some will eat dairy produce that is free of animal fat (e.g. cottage cheese). There are rules, such as eating with the right hand, and avoiding contact (touching) with other people's food. Swaminarayans also drink no coffee or alcohol, do not smoke, and eat no garlic or onions.

There are some days of the week when Hindus avoid eating specific foods and on certain days they may fast - which means eating 'pure' foods (i.e. fruit, yogurt) rather than starving.

The importance of food is such that some Hindus may refuse any food or even water outside their home. Ancient Hindu medicine (Ayurveda) places great emphasis on certain foods in maintaining health.

Main Languages
Gujurati and Hindi.

Ideas of Modesty
Modesty is important to Hindus; same-gender HCPs should be used where possible.

Attitudes to Healthcare Professionals
These are generally positive.

Health and Healing Traditions
Most Hindus do not perceive any great dichotomy between the Eastern and Western medical belief systems. There is a widespread respect for HCPs, who are considered to hold a high position in society. The patient may expect the doctors to have all the answers and make all the decisions and, as a result, may take a passive role, accepting advice without question. It is important to note, however, that mental illness is considered a stigma, so it is frequently concealed. Elderly patients may be stoic in expression of pain: it is important to observe non-verbal behaviour.

If the Western treatment fails to bring immediate relief of the symptoms, the patient may seek the care of a traditional physician or healer. Ayurveda is one of the oldest systems of traditional medicine, but others include homoeopathy, Unani, Siddha, yoga and naturopathy.

Hindus are also supposed not to drink alcohol or take drugs that affect the mind.

Some patients, in particular those who follow vegan or vegetarian diets, may object to the use of animals to meet the needs of humans. Donation of blood and organs is not usually restricted.

Oral Healthcare Issues
While routine dental care is accepted, the use of animal products, including gelatin in orabase and mucin in salivary substitutes, should be avoided, together with the use of products containing alcohol.

Relevant Websites
http://www.hindunet.org/ (The Hindu Universe: a large amount of information about Hinduism and associated topics.)

http://www.katha.org/Academics/Advaita-FrontPg.html (Advaita for Beginners: an online text on Hindu beliefs.)

Islam

Background

Muhammad (Mohammed), born in Saudi Arabia, at Mecca (Makkah) in AD 570, was the final prophet rather than founder of Islam. Mecca is the main shrine. Muhammad later migrated from Mecca to Medina to avoid persecution, an event known as hijra (Hegira or Hajj). The Islamic calendar begins at the time of the Hajj.

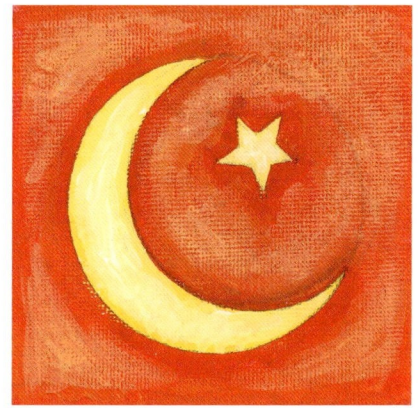

Islam is the world's second largest religion. It is the major religion in the Middle East and north Africa, and most Arabs are followers of Islam, i.e. Muslims. Islam is also the major religion in other parts of Africa – especially Nigeria – and in Central and South Asia, – in particular Indonesia, Pakistan, Bangladesh and India. In Europe, Islam is a major religion in Albania, much of the former Yugoslavia, Bulgaria, Turkey, France, Germany and the UK.

Beliefs

The word 'Islam' means submission and peace and obedience. Muslims believe that all human beings will ultimately be judged by God for their beliefs and actions in their earthly lives and that all events are God's will (insha'Allah – God willing – is a commonly used expression) and they submit to the will of God, regardless of their race, nationality or ethnic background.

Practical Islam (Din) consists of five observances (or pillars of wisdom), viz:
• Shahada (declaration of faith) – recital of the formula of belief
• Salah – prayer (see below)
• Saum – fasting during the period of Ramadan from dawn to sunset.
• Almsgiving – giving up a share of wealth each year to provide for those less fortunate.
• Hajj (pilgrimage) – having a duty to make a pilgrimage to the Ka'aba in Mecca at least once during their lifetime.

Islam consists of two main groups or branches. By far the larger group (85%) is the Sunni Muslims. Sunni comes from the Arabic word Sunna, meaning 'tradition'. Sunnis tend to stress merit and achievement.

The other group are the Shi'ites. The Shi'ites (from the Arabic word Shia, meaning 'partisan') are primarily found in Iran and Iraq and tend to appeal more to the defeated, poor and oppressed. Within each of the two branches there are various subgroups, each with its own conception of the nature of religious authority and the norms for lifestyle.

An individual Muslim's beliefs and practices may vary depending on the type of Islam he or she follows.

Culture
Muslim religion and culture are inextricably linked. Islam regulates all aspects of Muslim life, and the Islamic symbol – the moon and star - signifies how Islam guides and lights a Muslim's way through life. Muslims also believe strongly in the immortal soul and life after death.

Islam's sacred book is the Qur'an (Koran). All Muslims can read Arabic as in the Qur'an, and many speak it, but not all can.

Muslims aim to be just, compassionate, honest, generous, humble, patient and brave. Family life is central to Islam, and major duties include obedience to parents and care and respect for elders. Divorce is strongly disapproved of. Modesty is important, as outlined below.

Most men use a religious name (e.g. Mohammed) which comes first, or Ullah, which usually follows another name, but these religious names should not be used alone, rather with the second (or personal) name (e.g. Abdullah).

Worship
Prayers with ablution are made at five set times a day. This may be in the place of worship – a mosque (Fig 2-11), or anywhere, but always facing towards Mecca (Fig 2-12). Before prayer, Muslims should wash their hands, face and feet in running water.

Holy Days and Festivals
Friday is the Muslim holy day, and lunchtime prayers are especially important. There are two important holy days each year:
• Eid ul-Fitr (Id al-Fitr) – the festival of breaking the fast of Ramadan, a one-day celebration that falls on the first day of Shawwal, the month after Ramadan.
• Eid ul-Adha (Id al-Adha or Byram) – celebrated at the end of the Hajj

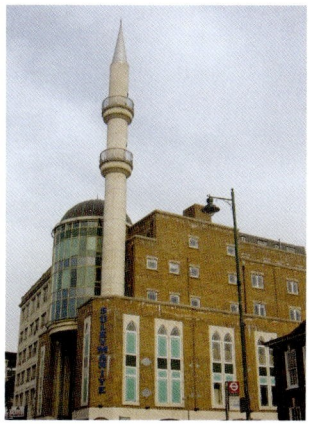 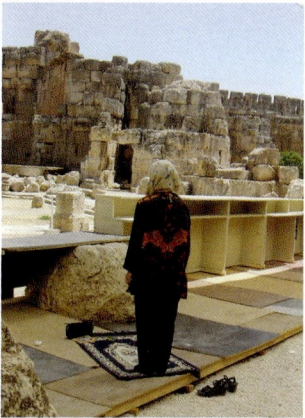

Fig 2-11 A main London mosque.

Fig 2-12 Muslim woman preparing for prayers in the Middle East.

(season of pilgrimage to Makkah) beginning on the 10th day of the month of Dhul Hijjah. Dates of the festivals are based on the lunar calendar and vary accordingly.

• Ramadan is the ninth month of the Islamic calendar, when there is fasting from dawn to sunset, which requires total abstinence from food, drink and tobacco, except for the sick, the elderly, children below the age of puberty, those on a long journey and pregnant women.

• Al-Hijra is the Islamic New Year.

Dietary and Other Habits and Restrictions

The general principle of Shariah (Muslim law) is that all food and drink is permitted (i.e. Halal) to Muslims, unless there is an explicit prohibition. Halal foods are prepared in specific ways (Figs 2-13 and 2-14). Pakistanis are especially strict.

Forbidden food and drink are termed haraam. For example, Muslims eat nothing that is from a pig, such as pork, ham, bacon and sausages, nor anything made from pork lard such as ice-cream or biscuits. Some shellfish are prohibited, as are fish without scales or fins. Alcohol and the use of illicit drugs are strictly forbidden.

Many Muslims away from home adopt a vegetarian diet in order to avoid foods that might contain non-halal products (e.g. gelatin, animal fat).

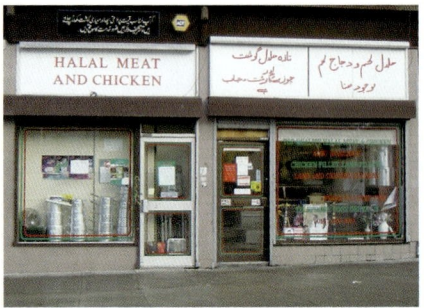

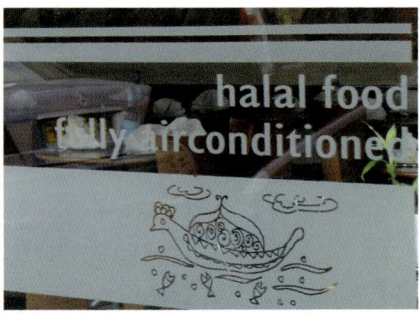

Fig 2-13 Shop offering Halal food in Scotland.

Fig 2-14 Restaurant offering Halal food in London.

Main Languages
Arabic, Bengai, Farsi, Gujarati, Hausa, Malay, Punjabi, Pushto, Sylheti, Turkish, Urdu.

Ideas of Modesty
Modesty in all aspects of Muslim life is important, for both men and women. The prescription for modesty is most evident among observant Muslim women who must cover themselves from head to toe with the exception of hands and face, often wearing a long tunic over loose trousers and the traditional head shawl (Fig 2-15). Women wear a hijab or head covering in public, which varies from a headscarf to a robe that covers the hair, neck and body, leaving the face and hands visible. There is great variety worldwide in the requirements for covering and the style of covering that is acceptable.

The clothes should neither be transparent nor reveal the shape of the woman's body. Shi'ite Muslim women dress typically in black, especially older women and widows, in full 'purdah' covering their bodies and faces. In western countries some Muslim women wear western dress, but they typically still dress modestly.

Muslim men from some traditions wear a kufi (a small cap), and others regard the wearing of a beard as a religious requirement. Muslim men must cover their bodies between the waist and knees, even when swimming or showering in public. Some wear a cap (tigiyah) especially for prayers (Fig 2-16).

Males and females do not touch in public. Segregation of the sexes (purdah) is the norm in some communities such as Shi'ites, in which women are not permitted to be alone with a man who is not her husband or relative (Fig 2-

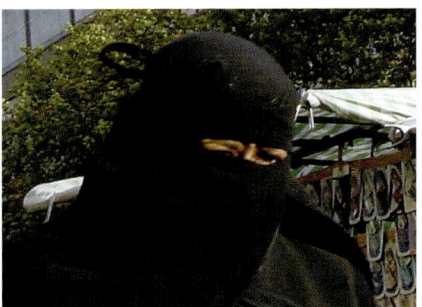 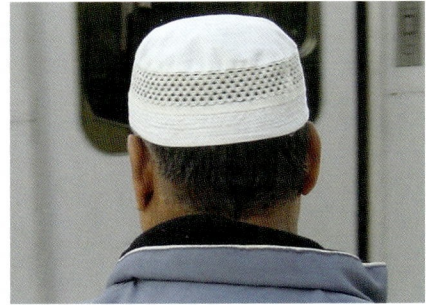

Fig 2-15 Muslim head covering.   **Fig 2-16** Tigiyah.

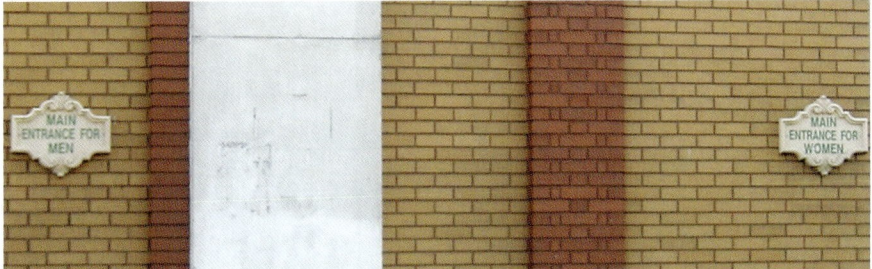

Fig 2-17 Mosque: separate entrances for each gender.

17). Thus in some Shi'ite communities, men and women are never in contact with someone of the opposite gender who is not from their family. It is never acceptable for a man to shake the hand of a Shi'ite woman. Handshakes are appropriate only between men or between women. The right hand is considered clean, and is used for eating, handshaking, and the like. Muslims may shake hands or embrace depending on the intimacy of the relationship.

Modesty in healthcare is very important. Muslim women may prefer female HCPs. A Shi'ite woman in particular may need to be treated by a female HCP and may refuse to be touched by a male.

For Muslims, interpreters of the same sex as the patient facilitate communication between patient and physician. If a same-sex interpreter is not available, and if there is concern that the female patient is not responsive because

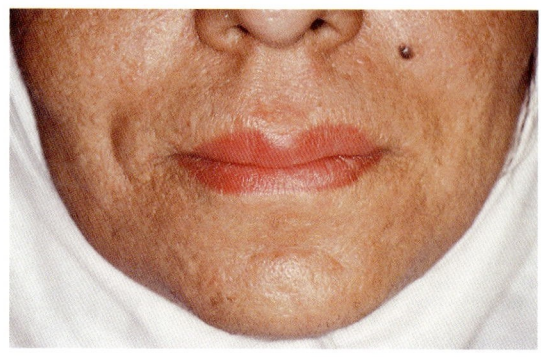

Fig 2-18 Hijab.

she is uncomfortable with a male interpreter, an alternative would be for the interpreter not to be visible to the patient or to interpret by telephone or speaker phone.

Some Muslims may not feel comfortable disclosing detailed information about themselves and their families to strangers. Personal questions can be embarrassing to them, and may be avoided unless the answers are needed by the HCP. Muslim men may not feel comfortable discussing problems, or even acknowledging the existence of problems, with a stranger, especially with a woman. They may try to give as little information as possible, and this may make diagnosis difficult.

Attitudes to Healthcare Professionals
These are generally positive.

Health and Healing Traditions
Muslims are strongly inclined to seek medical care and treatment. The health of each individual is of concern to the family as a whole, and therefore Muslim men frequently accompany their wives and children to appointments. Modesty is important, as discussed above, and the wearing of the hijab can impede full inspection and examination of the head and neck (Figs 2-18). Careful discussion and consent is required in examining and providing treatment.

Muslims may wish to avoid appointments on holy days and at prayer times, and particularly, some may wish treatment to be avoided on Fridays (especially at and after lunchtime prayers) and during Ramadan. Despite the fast of Ramadan (see above), treatment can be provided if necessary, but is best given after sunset. Prepubertal children, pregnant women and people with chronic illnesses or who must take medication regularly throughout the day are not obliged to fast during Ramadan but may wish so to do. Islam exempts sick people from fasting. However, many ill patients still decide to observe the fast. Fasting in any individual may produce a tendency to hypoglycaemia and irritability. Drugs, if needed, are best given orally once a day after sunset, or the patient may accept injections. Those with acute or serious conditions may need advice about altering the amount and frequency of their medication or their route of administration. Drugs that normally are required to be taken frequently, such as antibiotics, can be problematic, so drugs with long half-lives or sustained release preparations should be chosen. Azithromycin and doxycycline, for example, need to be taken only once daily. Alternative routes of drug administration such as transdermal (skin) patches of glyceryl trinitrate, rather than sublingual tablets, for angina pectoris may help.

Some Muslims prefer not to donate blood during Ramadan, but otherwise blood transfusion and donation are not an issue. Organ donation is halal, but there is often reluctance.

Oral Healthcare Issues
Muslims clean their teeth before prayers, often with the miswak. Western healthcare including dental care is accepted, although some Muslim men, who through humility avoid wearing gold jewelry and other items, may decline the use of gold in dental restorations.

There may be non-compliance with oral medication during fasts and it may therefore be best to avoid elective procedures where, for example, oral analgesics or antibiotics may be required, or to change to less-frequent oral dose regimens or to parenteral drugs. Where possible, dental treatment is best deferred until after sunset, or even until after Ramadan. Some Muslims may be concerned that the use of a local anaesthetic amounts to an intake of fluid, and many get concerned at the possibility of swallowing water from a three-in-one syringe. Some even worry about placing a toothbrush in their mouth. Toothpaste use is allowed during fasting (as long as it is not swallowed). The use of local and general anesthesia and/or sedation is allowed. During fasting, any individual has an increased liability to oral malodour.

There may be concerns that medicines and materials used are halal. The use of materials, products or devices (e.g. bristle polishing brushes), which contain animal products, in particular anything from the pig, should be avoided. This may extend to E numbers derived from porcine products and emulsifiers derived from animals. Queries can be directed to The Muslim Council of Britain, which runs a community information service 'MCB Direct'(www.mcb.org.uk/mcbdirect).

There is also concern with the use of alcohol in mouthwashes; alcohol-free oral products are better used, but alcohol-containing preparations are permitted if there is no alternative. Conditional use of alcohol containing medicines according to Islamic guidelines and practice is as follows:
• Any medicine/product containing alcohol (such as mouthwashes) is used to rinse with only, and consequently no swallowing, or ingestion or drinking is typical. It should be spat out and the mouth should be rinsed with water if necessary.
• If there is any therapeutic alternative to alcohol-containing medicines/products, then the alcohol-free alternative should be preferred and used.
• The therapeutic use of alcohol-containing medicines/products is permitted until the desired effect /treatment/cure is achieved.
• Any medicine/product containing alcohol that does not sedate, does not make someone drunk or intoxicated, is allowed until the desired/required therapeutic effect/cure is achieved.

Unnecessary or prolonged use of alcohol-containing medicines/products is not allowed or permitted, as there is a possibility of addiction or substance abuse (Consensus Statement from a round-table meeting with leading dental specialists in the Muslim community, December 13, 2004, London).

Relevant Websites
http://www.mcb.org.uk (Muslim Council of Britain)

http://www.muslim-answers.org/(Information and discussions about Islam in present day society)

Jainism
Background
Jainism, one of the oldest religions, contains many elements similar to Hinduism and Buddhism. It is almost entirely located in people from India.

Beliefs

Jains do not believe in a supreme or creator God. They honour 24 teachers (Tirthankaras) who enlightened the world with true nature of the universe and showed the true path to Salvation, especially Mahavira - the last Tirthankara.

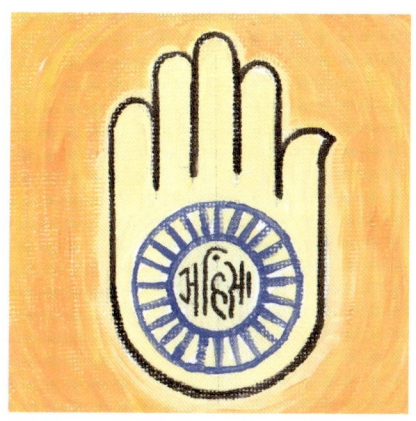

Jainism promotes righteousness and good moral and ethical practices and believes in equality of all human beings, regardless of caste, colour and creed, and respects and reveres womanhood. There is a clear code of dutiful and correct behaviour, of non-violence and compassion, and of seeking the truth. Jains practice Ahimsa - non violence, non-injury and non-killing - and believe that committing an act of violence against a human, animal, or even vegetable generates negative karma. Animal welfare, vegetarianism and care of the environment are therefore important in Jainism.

Culture

Major duties include obedience to parents and care and respect for elders. Family is central to Jainism and divorce is strongly disapproved of. Chastity and sexual continence are important.

Worship

Jains worship three times each day – morning, noon and sunset and at the beginning and end of the day, when they may 'retreat' for 48 minutes and be uncontactable.

Holy Days and Festivals

These include:
- Mahavira Jayanti – April
- Paryusana parva – August/September
- Diwali – October/November.

Dietary and Other Habits and Restrictions

- Jains are strict vegetarians: they eat no meat, fish or eggs, nor any prepared food containing these products or their derivatives or additives. Some Jains also avoid all root vegetables (including carrots, potatoes, onions, garlic),

butter, cheese, figs and honey (since any of these may contain micro-organisms). They do not approve of food prepared unsegregated from restricted foods. They do not drink alcohol or use tobacco. However, they usually drink milk.
- Some Jains fast on the fifth and 14th of each lunar month, and for the week of the Paryusana-parva.

Main languages
Bengali, Punjabi, Hindi, Gujarati, Tamil, Telugu.

Ideas of Modesty
This is important, as are same-gender HCPs.

Attitudes to Healthcare Professionals
These are generally positive.

Health and Healing Traditions
Endurance and self-discipline are important to Jains, and spiritual practices and human support more important than drugs. Jains may also, because of the prohibition on harming any form of life (including bacteria), refuse to take antibiotics. They may also be reluctant to take opiates. Some patients, particularly those who follow vegan or vegetarian diets, may object to the use of animals to meet the needs of humans, and therefore the use of animal products, including gelatin and mucin, should be avoided. Some Jains will not consume any root vegetables or their derivatives, which may preclude some E numbers used as colourants, e.g. carotene E160a. There are no problems related to blood transfusions or organ donations or receipts.

Oral Healthcare Issues
Western healthcare, including dental care, is generally accepted. There is concern over the use of alcohol or animal products in mouthwashes and related products.

Relevant Website
http://www.jainworld.com/ (Jainism Global Resource Centre)

Judaism

The Mager David – the Star of David, is the symbol most commonly associated with Judaism.

Background

Judaism is a very old religion. According to Judaism, Christianity and Islam, both the Jews and the Arabs are descended from patriarch Abraham: Jews are the descendants of Isaac through Jacob and Arabs are the descendants of Ishmael. Jews (from Judah), originally descendants of Judah, the fourth son of Jacob, whose tribe, with that of his half-brother Benjamin, made up the kingdom of Judah.

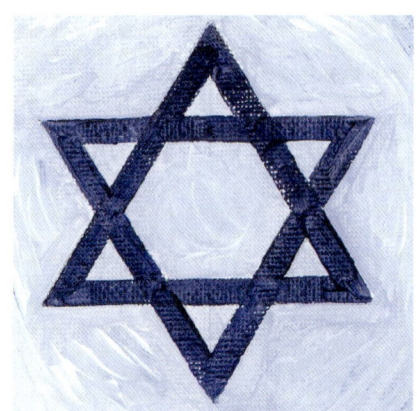

The Roman occupation of the Jewish homeland in Israel resulted in some Jews emigrating to Portugal and Spain, and others were taken to Rome as captives, migrating from there to western Europe and Scandinavia. The Sephardim, a branch of Judaism arising from descendants of these Spanish and Portuguese Jews, are spread throughout the Mediterranean world and western Europe.

The other large branch (Ashkenazim), originated in the Rhine valley and migrated east into Poland and Russia. There they used to speak Yiddish, a German-Jewish language.

Judaism is centered on the City of Jerusalem. Although generally considered a major religion, the Jewish people only make up 0.23% of the world population. In 2005, there were approximately 15 million Jews in the world – eight million in the Americas, 3.5 million in Israel, and 3.5 million in Europe.

Beliefs

Jews believe they were promised by God (often written G-d) to be the chosen people and that God would lead and protect them until they reached the Kingdom Of Heaven. Jews believe that there is a single God who not only created the universe, but with whom every Jew can have an individual and personal relationship and who continues to work in the world, affecting everything that people do. The Jewish relationship with God is regarded as a 'covenant' relationship.

Most Jews belong to a synagogue (shul), a meeting place where Jews read the Torah and pray, and in which the religious leader is the Rabbi (teacher),

97

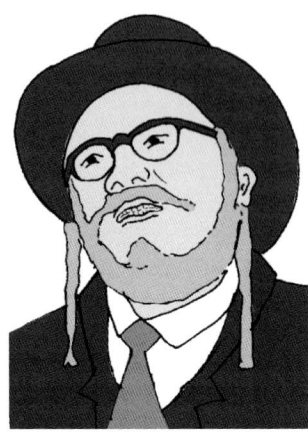

Fig 2-19 An orthodox Jewish man.

who is also a guide and pastor to the synagogue community. One day each week is set aside as the Sabbath ('Shabbat'), the Jewish holy day. Shabbat starts just before sunset on Friday and ends at nightfall on Saturday.

There are a number of Jewish traditions. The most important division is between 'orthodox' (Hasidic, Haredim), conservative (Masorti) and 'reform' and 'liberal' Jews, with many subdivisions, and then there are 'secular Jews'.

Orthodox Judaism
Orthodox Jews tend to take their holy days and fasting seriously. Daily attendance at the synagogue is encouraged. On Shabbat, orthodox Jews carry out no work and avoid carrying anything outside the home, driving, using transport, handling money, cooking, writing, or signing papers, or using gas or electricity in any way (including the telephone, fax, internet and email). Some will not open post or packages, tear paper, use creams or ointments, or alter the shape of anything (e.g. they may avoid using toothpaste, and prefer to use a tooth powder).

Many Orthodox men always keep their heads covered and wear a fringed garment (tsitsit) under their shirt. Some wear their hair in side locks (Fig 2-19). Ultra-orthodox women outside the house cover their heads with a wig (sheitel) or scarf and wear high necklines, long sleeves and skirts below the knees.

Touch between an Orthodox woman and man is forbidden unless they are married and, although this is waived for medical purposes, same-gender

HCPs are preferred. Nevertheless, orthodox people of opposite genders should not be alone in a room together and should not touch unnecessarily, even to shake hands.

Reform/Liberal/Progressive Movements
These Jews, chiefly prevalent in the UK and the United States, believe that individuals can make choices about what traditions to follow, and they tend to disregard dietary laws, second days of festivals, minor feasts, and fast-days except Hanukkah and Purim.

Secular Jews are people who call themselves Jews but do not believe in all aspects of the religion – rather they think of their Jewishness as a matter of culture or ethnicity, of identity with the state of Israel, of the food, of some limited holy day observances, and of cultural values like the emphasis on education. Probably about half of all Jews in the United States, for example, fall into this category.

Culture
Jewish religion and culture are inextricably linked. Jews are life-affirming and generally disciplined, hard-working, entrepreneurial and family-orientated. Loyalty to host countries is a religious principle. Judaism generally places high value on study and intellectual understanding, questioning and analysis.

The Jewish naming system is a first name and a surname, but Jews also have a Hebrew name for use in Synagogue and on religious documents.

Worship
Male Jews are meant to attend the synagogue for prayer three times daily (morning, afternoon, and evening), or to say their prayers in privacy at home. Blessings and praises of thanksgiving are also recited before and after meals and on other occasions. Jewish men wear a hat or skull cap called a kippah (Yarmulke) when at prayer or the synagogue. Some Jews wear a kippah all of the time as a mark of respect for God (Fig 2-20).

For Orthodox Jews, in their morning devotions, men use phylacteries (tefillin) – two small boxes attached to leather straps - and a prayer scarf (tallit), except on Saturdays, when they use the tallit only.

Holy Days and Festivals
Saturday is set aside as the Sabbath ('Shabbat'), the Jewish holy day. Shabbat starts just before sunset on Friday with the lighting of Shabbat candles and a

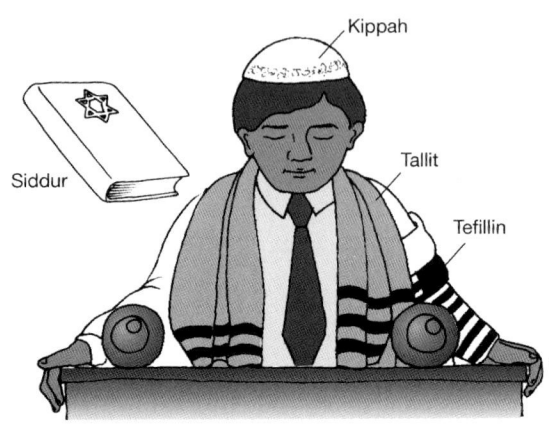

Fig 2-20 Jewish worship.

family supper, ending at nightfall on Saturday with a ceremony called Havdalah.

Shabbat is a day devoted to family time as well as prayer, religious study, relaxation and refreshment. Work, including shopping and cleaning, must be avoided, in particular by orthodox Jews, but some Jews keep their businesses open because of commercial demands. Treatment should normally be avoided on Shabbat, but emergencies override the various restrictions.

Important celebrations during which treatment should be avoided include:
- Pesach – the start of Passover is in March/April. The first two and last days are observed as strict holidays.
- Shavuot – Pentecost is the time when the Jews received God's laws (Torah) at Mount Sinai. Lasts for two days, which are observed as strict holy days and falls in May/June.
- Tish'ah B'Av – the second holiest fast day of the year which is a 25-hour fast and commemorates the destruction of the Temple in Jerusalem. Normally falls in late July/August.
- Rosh Hashana – the Jewish equivalent of what Christians call New Year's Day is a strict two-day festival in September or October.
- Yom Kippur – the holiest day of the Jewish year, is a strict 25-hour fast that falls eight days after Rosh Hashana. Not even water must pass the lips.
- Succot – a nine-day harvest festival – the Feast of Tabernacles. The first two and last two days are observed as strict holy days – September/October.

• Hanukkah – the 'Festival of Lights' – celebrated by the lighting of candles and the preparation of potato cakes. This festival lasts eight days. In Christian countries where Christmas is the major festival, Hanukkah has become the Jewish equivalent. Hanukkah starts early to mid-December. Most Jews will attend for routine treatment during Hanukkah, as these are not strict holydays.

Dietary and Other Habits and Restrictions

Observant Jews eat only food that is kosher (slaughtered and prepared according to Jewish law). Kosher (permitted) foods and drink are prepared in specific ways and care has to be taken not to contaminate the prepared food with treifah (non-kosher) foods and cooking utensils.

Pork, shellfish or predatory fowl or products made from them are forbidden (non-kosher), as are fish without scales or fins. These observances may extend to avoiding animal fats or products in other foods, medications etc. Thus jellies (which contain gelatin) and cheese (which contains animal rennet) are usually unacceptable. Meat and milk, or their products, are not cooked together or eaten at the same meal.

Wine and grape juice are permitted but must come from a rabbinically approved source. Even where the ingredients are acceptable, the product may still be non-kosher because of agents used in its manufacture. The London Beth Din *Really Jewish Food Guide* is a widely used guide (Fig 2-21).

Jews fast on several days during the year, with the most important fast days being Tish'ah B'Av and especially Yom Kippur. During Pesach, Jews do not eat foods containing flour or yeast.

Main Languages

These depend on country of origin.

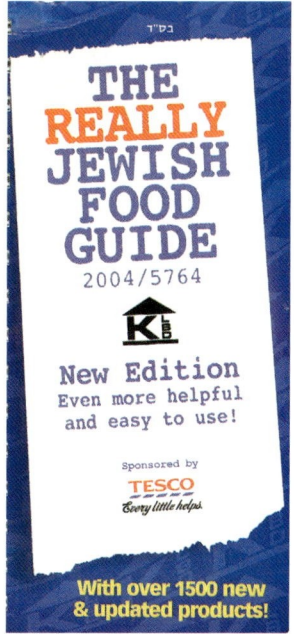

Fig 2-21 Jewish food guide.

101

Ideas of Modesty
For the treatment of orthodox Jews, in particular, same-gender HCPs are favoured; opposite genders should not touch unnecessarily, even to shake hands; and privacy is important. The head should be kept covered.

Attitudes to Healthcare Professionals
Jews typically are very positive.

Health and Healing Traditions
Western healthcare, including dental care, is widely accepted and favoured. Medical issues in Judaism are subject not to a concept of Jewish medical ethics, but rather to the concept of Jewish medical law as contained in the halachic codes.

Treatment should normally be avoided on Shabbat or other holy days, but emergencies can over-ride the various restrictions.

HCPs need to be aware that many commonly available medicaments contain animal products that are forbidden to Jews. In medicines the issues are often with the excipients, rather than the active ingredients. Problem excipients may include:

- *Gelatin*: this is usually of animal origin, and not permitted. However, where it is being consumed in a non-edible form - for example, a totally tasteless capsule shell or a powdered form as a binder in tablets - it would be permitted if no alternative were readily available.
- *Glycerin*: can be of animal or vegetable origin. Almost all glycerin now used by the pharmaceutical industry is of vegetable extraction, and thus acceptable. Glycerin of animal origin is unacceptable and that in a liquid preparation would be forbidden as it helps to impart a good taste.
- *Stearic acid/stearates*: likewise are now usually from vegetable sources. There would also not be an issue if the preparation were a non-edible tablet.
- *Lactose*: a milk-derived sugar found in a wide range of tablets as a bulking agent and also used to make tablets that are chewable or suckable taste better is precluded. The issues are with respect to dietary laws that preclude consumption of milk and meat together and requirements for the supervision of milk. Alternatives should be sought with respect to edible products – for example, lactulose. Where the product is inedible, it is acceptable and reassurance should be given.

There can be, however, be some misunderstanding of treatments that are permitted under Jewish Law (Halacha). Pesach can present problems relating to medicines that contain wheat starch, since Jews are forbidden then to eat anything that contains flour that has risen.

Any medication can be taken even if it conflicts with dietary laws as long as no suitable alternative exists. Furthermore, in principle, the saving of life takes precedence over any law and, during times of illness, porcine-derived medicines and materials (for example) may be temporarily exempt, but exemption needs to be determined by the Rabbi. In the event of any uncertainty about the acceptability of a preparation, the patient should be consulted and advice sought, as considered necessary from the local Rabbi. The 'Shulchan Oruch. Yoreh Deah' 33 (The Code of Jewish Law) contains guidance on forbidden substances; translations for the non-Jewish reader can be obtained via 'Hakohol Kashrus' - a general guide to Kosher products, including medicines.

Jews have a strong belief in the sanctity of life. Donation and receipt of blood are widely accepted, but approval for organ donation or receipt will generally be dependent on the community Rabbi. Many Jewish authorities permit the withholding of heroic, life-prolonging intervention, other than food and fluids, for those whose are terminally ill, but no euthanasia is accepted.

Home/traditional medicine is rarely used and anecdotal in nature. It is widely believed, however, that traditional 'chicken soup' has medicinal powers, with a side-product (sodium cytarabine hexamethyl-acetyl lututria tetrazolamine) produced during its preparation possibly reducing the opportunity for pathogens to damage the nasal lining and, as such, may be efficacious in the management of upper respiratory infections.

Oral Healthcare Issues
Oral hygiene and tooth brushing are avoided on Shabbat and fast days. Shabbat restrictions on work (a creative act or acts which change one condition into another) could affect the wearing of orthodontic headgear and removable appliances. Routine treatment and, in particular, surgery should be avoided on holy days and festivals as well as Shabbat (Friday evenings and Saturdays).

Within strictly orthodox communities there are concerns over having temporary restorations (fillings and crowns) and the immersion of dentures to cleanse food and plaque at times of Pesach. There are a number of single-day festivals within the Jewish calendar that involve fasting. The stricter of these (Yom Kippur and Tish'ah B'Av) forbid a patient to take anything into their mouth. If oral analgesics are needed, it may not be permissible to take them with water. Animal-containing products such as gelatin (in Orabase and some medication capsules) and mucin (in some salivary substitutes such as Saliva Orthana) should be avoided, in particular when suitable alternatives exist. There may be concerns over the use of alcohol in mouthwashes.

Relevant Websites

http://www.jewfaq.org/ (Judaism 101 is an online encyclopedia of Judaism, covering Jewish beliefs, people, places, things, language, scripture, holidays, practices and customs)

http://www.jewishnet.net/ (Global Jewish Information Network)

http://www.kosher.org.uk/what.htm (Kosher food information from the London Beth Din Kashrut Division)

Paganism

The Pentagram has magical associations, and many people who practise pagan faiths wear it. Christians once commonly used the pentagram to represent the five wounds of Jesus, but nowadays some associate the symbol with Satanism.

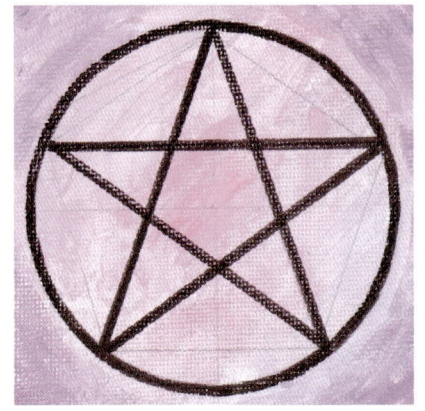

Background

Paganism is a collection of diverse contemporary religions rooted in or inspired by indigenous traditions rather than someone who is not a Christian, Muslim, or Jew. Examples include Asatru, Celticism, Church of All Worlds, Druidism, Odinism, Shamanism and Witchcraft (Wicca).

Beliefs

Pagans look to the beliefs, practices, gods, symbols, lands, music, and myths of a particular historical culture and adapt them for contemporary needs, retaining elements such as reverence for the natural world, honouring of ancestors, and responsibility to the community, but rejecting elements such as ritual violence. Pagans view all living things as sacred and they value diversity, good works, individual freedom, personal responsibility, community service, gender equity and spiritual development. Some Pagans are animists (they believe that personalised supernatural beings [or souls] inhabit all objects and govern their existence).

Holy Days and Festivals
Most Pagan religions follow the Wheel of the Year for celebrations, holy days and festivals. Names and exact dates may vary. Some traditions celebrate only the solstices and equinoxes. Observance of festivals is important to Pagans.

Dietary and Other Habits and Restrictions
Many Pagans are vegetarian and some are vegans. Many of those who do eat meat will object to meat from intensively farmed stock.

Main languages
Language depends on country.

Ideas of Modesty
There is no special issue.

Attitudes to Healthcare Professionals
Generally positive, albeit somewhat guarded by some.

Health and Healing Traditions
There are no special issues.

Oral Healthcare Issues
Avoid products of animal origin when treating, in particular, vegans.

Relevant Website
http://www.bloomington.in.us/pen/mpagan.html (Pagan Educational Network: information about paganism.)

Rastafarianism

Background

Invented by an American (Marcus Garvey) in Jamaica in the 1920s, as a backlash against white domination, Rastafarianism is a Bible-based, Christianised religion founded on the belief that Haile Selassie I, Emperor of Ethiopia (previously known as Ras Tafari Makonnen – The Lion of Judah), was the living God for the Black race. There are possibly one million Rastafarians worldwide. The overwhelming majority is of African ancestry, but there are also Chinese, East Indians, mixed, and a few whites.

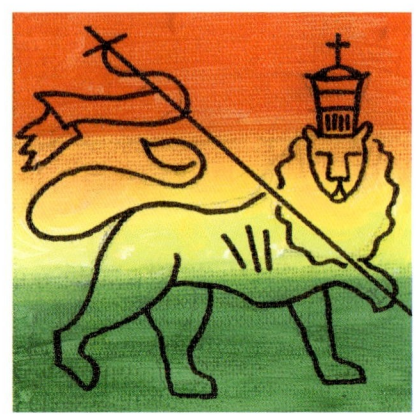

Beliefs

Rastafarians (Rastas) beliefs are similar to those of Christians. They may belong to a church and often use the Bible for guidance. Certain sections of the Bible are considered sacred, but Rastafarians believe that some aspects were changed by 'Babylon,' which has come to represent the white power structure. Many Rastafarians reject the Bible used by most Christians, opting instead for a 'black man's Bible,' known as the Holy Piby.

The Rasta name for God is Jah, and the 'livity' (way of life) is concerned with obeying Jah and recognition of Ethiopia as the New Jerusalem and spiritual homeland - the Promised Land. For Rastafarians there is no after-life or hell.

Many Rastafarians belong to the Twelve Tribes of Israel, an organisation with the philosophy to educate the young to help advancement of Black people, and the promotion of African and Ethiopian culture.

Culture

Rastafarians are typically of African descent, and grow their hair long and plait it in dreadlocks (Fig 2-22), often covered with a tam. Women are supposed to keep their hair covered with a tam or wrap. Reggae music is a feature of Rastafarian culture.

Holy Days and Festivals
The main Rastafarian holy days and festivals include:
- Ethiopian Christmas – January
- Birthday of Haile Selassie – July
- New Year's Day – September

In general, it is best to avoid treatment at these times.

Dietary and Other Habits and Restrictions
Devoted Rastafarians are vegetarian and eat only I-tal food – which is organic. The food is cooked, but served in the rawest form possible, without salts, preservatives or condiments. Most Rastafarians never eat pork and most do not eat fish with scales. Alcohol, milk, coffee and soft drinks are viewed as unnatural: anything that is herbal, such as tea or cannabis, is preferred.

Main languages
Rastas talk Patois, a Caribbean slang, or English and some learn Amharic, the Ethiopian national language.

Ideas of Modesty
There are no special issues.

Attitudes to Healthcare Professionals
HCPs are generally accepted.

Health and Healing Traditions
Some patients, particularly those who follow vegan or vegetarian diets, may object to the use of animals to meet the needs of humans. Some Rastas may refuse blood transfusions or organ donations.

Oral Healthcare Issues
The use of animal products, in particular porcine products, should be avoided. Examples include gelatin (in

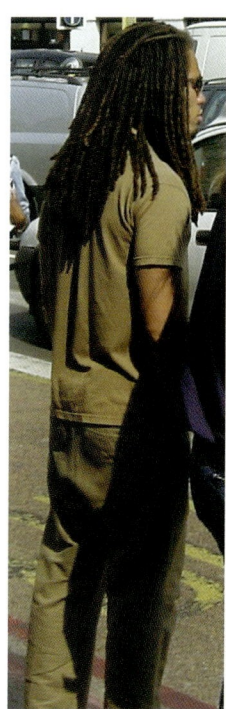

Fig 2-22 Rastafarian.

Orabase) and mucin in salivary substitutes. Otherwise the provision of routine care should not pose any difficulties.

Relevant Website
http://www.watchman.org/profile/rastapro.htm

Shintoism

Background
Shintoism is the religion encompassing rituals and customs that began in Japan during ancient times. The introduction of Buddhism and Confucianism to Japan in 552 AD prompted the adoption of the term 'Shinto'. There are almost three million proponents worldwide.

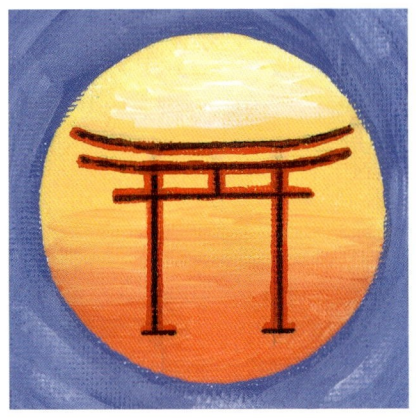

Beliefs
Shintoism is characterised by veneration of nature (all human life and human nature is considered sacred), spirits and ancestors and by a lack of formal dogma. Indeed, there is no scripture of Shintoism, but the Kojiki and Nihongi are comprehensive texts on the history of Japan and its mythology, wherein Shintoism has its roots.

Shinto recognizes various 'Kami', deities that serve only to sustain and protect, but has no body of religious law, and only a very loosely organised priesthood. Shintoism does not have a system of ethics or morals, but rather places emphasis on ritual and ceremony to express the joyful acceptance of nature. Shinto has no absolute rules outside of living 'a simple and harmonious life with nature and people', but the 'Four Affirmations' of the Shinto spirit include:
- Tradition and the family. Tradition and the family are very important. The family is seen as the main mechanism by which traditions are preserved. The main celebrations relate to birth and marriage.

- Love of nature. Nature is sacred, to be in contact with nature is to be close to the Kami. Natural objects are worshipped as containing sacred spirits.
- Physical cleanliness. Followers take baths, wash their hands and rinse their mouth often.
- 'Matsuri'. Any festival dedicated to the Kami should be celebrated.

Holy Days and Festivals
- Ganjitsu - New Year's Day – January
- O-Bon - Festival of Souls – July/August
- Omisoka – December.

Culture
The influence of Shinto on Japanese culture cannot be overestimated. It is still common for Japanese to say 'Itadakimasu' (I humbly partake) before eating, and the Japanese emphasis on proper greetings can be seen as a continuation of the ancient Shinto belief in kotodama (words with a magical effect on the world). Many Japanese cultural customs, including the use of wooden chopsticks and removing shoes before entering a building, have their origin in Shintoism.

Main Languages
Japanese.

Ideas of Modesty
There are no special issues.

Attitudes to Healthcare Professionals
There are no special issues.

Health and Healing Traditions
There are no special issues.

Oral Healthcare Issues
There are no special issues.

Relevant Websites
http://www.jinja.or.jp/english/(Shinto Online Network Association. - a non-profit volunteer organisation for publicising Japanese tradition and a correct understanding of the Shinto religion)

Sikhism

Background

Sikhism was founded in Punjab over 500 years ago by Shri Guru Nanak Devji, a Hindu teacher. He developed the new faith using ideas from both Hinduism and Islam, and based on the principles of one God and the equality of humans. Sikhism is centered on the holy City of Amritsar, where the sacred books of the faith are preserved and worshipped. Shikhism is a major religion in India and is ranked as the worlds fifth largest religion, with over 20 million Sikhs worldwide.

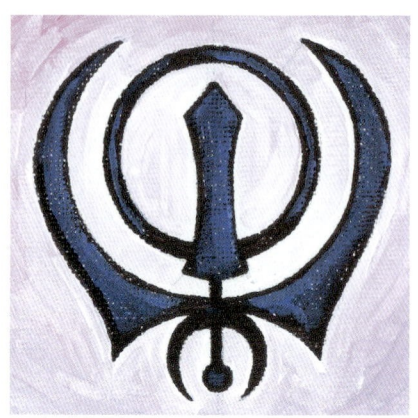

Beliefs

The essence of Sikhism is the belief in a single, formless God, with many names, who can be known through meditation. Sikhs also believe in samsara - the repetitive cycle of birth, life and death (reincarnation), and karma – the accumulative sum of one's good and bad deeds. The Gurdwara is the place used by the community, for worship and meeting.

Sikhs believe in living a responsible life as part of the community and the code of conduct – the Reht Maryada which condemns rituals including fasting, pilgrimages and worship of idols and the dead. Sikhs strive to earn an honest living, avoiding worldly temptations, with caring for the poor and the sick as an important duty of service. The essence of Sikh teaching is:
- There is only one God.
- Work hard and help others.
- Be honest.
- Everyone is equal in the eyes of God.
- Be kind to all, people and creatures.
- Fear nothing, pray for the good of all.
- Be simple and truthful in your daily life.

Khalsa are Sikhs who have undergone Sikh baptism, after which they are not permitted to:
- Remove hair from any part of the body

- Use tobacco, alcohol or any other intoxicants
- Eat meat.

Culture
Most Sikhs have three names: a personal name (which often can be used for either girls or boys, e.g. Balvinder), a name to show Sikh identity (Singh - meaning lion) and a clan or sub-sect name. Women often just use Kaur (princess) as a third name but can also use 'Singh', as many families have taken this as a surname.

Worship
Sikhs tend to pray at sunrise and sunset, typically washing beforehand. Sikhism does not have priests, hence services are led by any devout Sikh who can read the Guru Granth Sahib.

Holy Days and Festivals
Sunday is the day Sikhs tend not to work, but to worship - at the Gurdwara. The main festivals include:
- Vaisakhi (Baisakhi) - the Sikh New Year festival – April
- Gurpurbs - festivals associated with the lives of the Gurus (e.g. the Births of Guru Gobind Singh and Guru Nanak)
- Diwali - the Festival of Light – October
- Hola Mahalla - a festival of martial arts – March.

Dietary and Other Habits and Restrictions
Most Sikhs are vegetarian. Sikhs do not eat beef or any meat from animals which have been ritually slaughtered (halal, kosher): meat should be slaughtered according to the Sikh rite Jhatka. Baptised Sikhs are vegetarian and do not drink alcohol or coffee, or smoke. The staple food is bread (chapatti). Water or buttermilk (lasi) is drunk with meals. Sikhs rarely fast for religious reasons.

Main Languages
Punjabi is the main language.

Ideas of Modesty
Women prefer care by female HCPs. Sikh men neither cut their hair nor shave. The turban is used to cover the uncut hair and is mandatory for Sikh men (Figs 2-23 and 2-24) but optional for Sikh women who tend to cover their heads with a scarf (dupattah or chooni), when praying. It should not be covered by any other headgear or replaced by a cap or hat. Some women

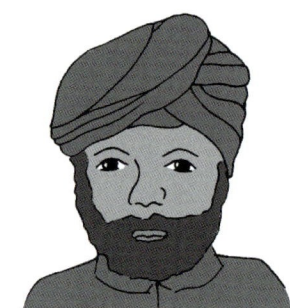

Fig 2-23 Turban.

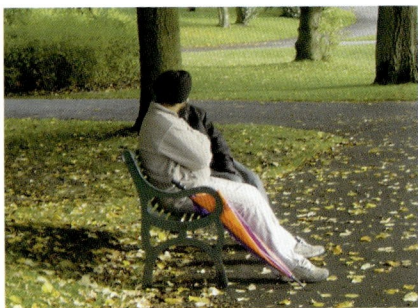

Fig 2-24 Sikh dress.

wear a small dot on their forehead (bindi) for decoration only. The traditional dress for women is a shalwar kameez (tunic and trousers). Men tend to wear Western-style trousers and shirt, although a kameez/kurtha (tunic) and pyjamas (traditional trousers) may be worn at home or to the Gurdwara.

If it is necessary to ask a Sikh to remove the turban, or other head covering in the case of Sikh women, an alternative cover, such as a surgical bouffant cap, should be provided. The turban or other head covering, if removed, should be respected and should never be placed with shoes. Where appropriate, it should be given to the family. A Khalsa Sikh must also wear the five 'K's:

- Kesh – uncut hair
- Kangha – a wooden comb
- Kara – a steel bracelet
- Kacha – loose, white, cotton undergarment
- Kirpaan – a ceremonial sword (nowadays tends to be a small replica).

These must not be disturbed without consent or unless absolutely necessary.

Attitudes to Healthcare Professionals
There are no special issues.

Health and Healing Traditions
Sikhs may tend to use home remedies and may be slow to seek professional attention. Sikhs regard caring for the poor and sick as an important duty of service. It is therefore important to be understanding of family members and friends who wish to attend together with a patient.

In general, it is best to avoid treatment at the time of the major Sikh festivals. Animal products in medicaments, e.g., gelatin and mucin should be avoided, but alcohol in prescribed products is usually acceptable, as the intention is not to intoxicate.

The patient, or parents or guardian in the case of a child, should be consulted prior to shaving or otherwise removing hair from any part of the patient's body, whether male or female. Where indicated clinically, hair removal is usually permitted. Permission should be sought and hands washed before touching the Guru Granth Sahib (holy book). The book must never be placed on the floor or close to someone's feet.

Receipt of blood, blood products, and organs is allowed: the Sikh religion teaches that life continues after death in the soul and not the physical body. The last act of giving and helping others through organ donation is both consistent with, and in the spirit of, Sikh teachings.

Oral Healthcare Issues
Acceptance of dental care is good. Sikhs have widespread respect for western healthcare, but may supplement prescribed medication with traditional therapies, including homoeopathic remedies.

Relevant Websites
http://allaboutsikhs.com/home.php (Complete Sikhism resource site)

http://www.bbc.co.uk/worldservice/people/features/world_religions/sikhism.shtml (BBC World Service guide to religion and ethics, Sikhism section.)

Taoism

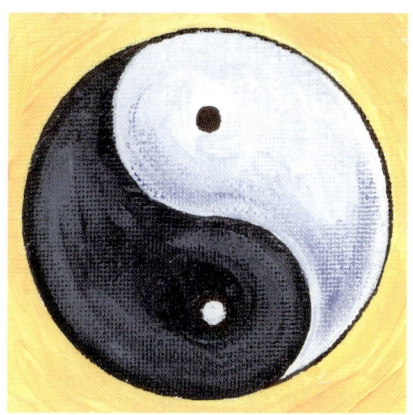

Background
Taoism is a major Chinese religion stemming largely from the Tao-te-ching, 'The Way of Power,' or 'The Book of the Way' – a text ascribed to the founder Lao Tzu. There are about 20 million Taoists worldwide.

Beliefs
Because the tradition is so ancient, and is linked so closely with Confucianism,

it can be difficult to distinguish the individual beliefs. Taoism is a polytheistic religion – there is not one single god to worship. Rather, Taoists seek the solutions to life's problems through meditation and observation. Taoism sees life as a balance of water, earth, fire, wood and metal and tries to achieve health, harmony and balance, and avoids disharmony and conflict. Tao philosophy in many ways advocates noninterference and inaction: learning to detach oneself from the world and allowing things to become what they will. This involves finding the 'way,' or 'tao', by 'flowing in accordance with nature' and remaining in harmony with both the cosmological (yin/yang) and natural spheres. Following the natural ebb and flow of the universe means that one adopts the chung-yung, or golden mean, by maintaining a middle position that avoids extremes.

The Taoist cyclical view of nature implies that one should remain in harmony with the changing of the seasons, the waxing and waning of the moon, and the rhythm of night and day. Taoism teaches that life, too, is a cycle consisting of birth, death, and reincarnation; that all things in nature ebb and flow, reaching one extreme (e.g. fortune) and then reverting to the other (e.g. misfortune).

Main languages
Chinese

Ideas of Modesty
See Chinese

Attitudes to Healthcare Professionals
See Chinese

Health and Healing Traditions
See Chinese

Asians instinctively show stoicism in the face of illness and danger, which should not be misunderstood by Westerners. Caregivers should make every effort to understand and respect these beliefs and attitudes.

There may be restrictions on donations or receipt of blood, blood products or organs.

Taoists undertake various exercise and movement techniques. Traditional Chinese medicine teaches that illness is caused by blockages or lack of balance in the body's 'chi' (intrinsic energy). Tai chi is believed to balance this energy flow and is said to works on all parts of the body as it 'stimulates the central nervous system, lowers blood pressure, relieves stress and gently tones muscles without strain. It also enhances digestion, elimination of wastes and the circulation of blood.'

Oral Healthcare Issues
As in Confucianism, attitudes towards western healthcare are similar to those found amongst Chinese (see Chinese). Most prefer traditional Chinese medicines in conjunction with western medicines.

Relevant Website
http://www.religioustolerance.org/falungong.htm (Information about Falun Gong and Falun Dafa in China and elsewhere. Also some information about Buddhism and Taoism)

Zoroastrianism

Background
Zoroastrianism was founded thou-sands of years ago, by Zarathushtra (Zoroaster), who lived in central Asia, possibly in Azerbaijan or Greater Iran, areas connected by a common Iranian culture and whose populations once commonly practised Zoroastrianism. Nowadays, aside from the Parsis of India, fewer than 10,000 persons practise Zoroastrianism, mainly in Iran, India, UK, North America and Aus-tralasia.

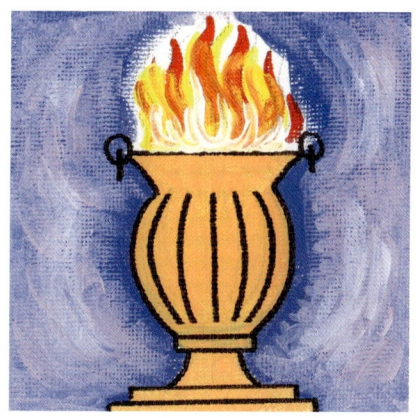

Beliefs
Zoroastrians worship through prayers and symbolic ceremonies that are conducted before the sacred fire, representing the light that gives all life. They dedicate their lives to 'good thoughts, good words, and good deeds'. There are two fundamental ideas in Zoroastrianism:
• free will and individual responsibility for one's own actions; and
• the concepts of good and evil.

The path of righteousness ('Asha') or purity in thought, word and deed will lead to happiness ('ushta') but the alternative choice – deceit, lies and unkindness, impurity of thought, word and deed – will lead to unhappiness, enmity and war. Their scripture is the Avesta.

Culture
Bodily cleanliness is important and the wearing of the white muslin undergarment, the 'sedreh', donned at the initiation ceremony of 'sedreh pushi', represents this. Zoroastrians do good deeds, including alms–giving. Parsis (Parsees), especially those raised in East Africa, tend to be orthodox.

Zoroastrians have three names; the forename, a middle name (father's forename) and surname (family name – which may indicate a profession).

Worship
Prayers are said in Pahlavi and Avesta, ancient Iranian languages. The place of worship is the Fire Temple.

Holy Days and Festivals
In general, try and avoid treatment on these.
- Nawroz (No Ruz or beginning of Spring) – March
- Khordad Sal (Fasli) – birth of the prophet Zarathrustra – March
- Zartusht – death of the prophet Zarathrustra – May
- Farsi New Year – August
- Zartusht (Zarthost)- No - Diso (Fasli) – December.

Dietary and Other Habits and Restrictions
The orthodox Zoroastrians eat no pork or beef, but these are not religiously restricted. Alcohol is permitted.

Main Languages
Parsi or English.

Ideas of Modesty
Zoroastrians should always wear the sudreh (a shirt) and kushti (cord wrapped around the waist). These should not be removed without consent.

Attitudes to Healthcare Professionals
There are no special issues.

Health and Healing Traditions
There are no special issues.

116

Oral Healthcare Issues
There are no special issues.

Relevant Website
http://www.w-z-o.org/ (The World Zoroastrian Organisation homepage)

http://www.beliefnet.com/index/index_10000.html (General information about major world religions and belief systems, with comparisons between them)

http://bible.gospelcom.net/bible (Bible Gateway.com A Ministry of Gospel Communications. Search system for finding passages in the Bible)

http://mcel.pacificu.edu/as/students/vb/Caodai.htm (Cao Dai. Short descriptions of this and other religions)

Section 3
Cultural Groups

Aim

This section presents outlines of various main cultural groups that may be encountered, giving an outline of their religions and languages, together with generalised information on dietary and other habits and restrictions, health and healing traditions and oral healthcare issues.

Outcome

This section should come to be viewed as a source of reference to enhance culturally sensitive healthcare through knowledge and understanding of different cultural groups.

Overview

Patients' views, reactions to illness, health needs and expectations of treatment vary widely and are influenced by many factors, of which cultural groups may be but one. Grouping diverse peoples leads to inevitable generalisations and sometimes can lead to errors and misunderstanding, but can often be a helpful guide, provided that all patients are treated as individuals.

Cultural convictions and beliefs may govern a patient's life or, at the other extreme, have limited, if any, influence on their views, needs and wishes. A patient's attitude towards their culture, its beliefs and practices may change with time.

Healthcare providers (HCPs) must be sensitive to such issues to best relate to patients and to avoid possible criticisms of insensitivity, let alone run the risk of giving offence. At all times patients must be treated as individuals, never stereotyped.

Certain cultural beliefs and practices may unfortunately be viewed as barriers to best possible clinical outcomes and thereby present the HCP with ethical problems. Such situations are best managed by carefully listening to the individual patient's needs, wishes and concerns, and through discussions between patient and HCPs as to how best to address possible conflicts and dilemmas.

The HCP must never make assumptions based on generalisations and thereby increase the risk of creating difficulties and causing offence.

In view of the enormous diversity in cultures and health beliefs and practices, it is only possible to discuss these from the traditional perspective as seen in the home country. Individuals may subscribe to all, some or none, and the only way to provide culturally sensitive healthcare is to be sensitive to each and every patient and, when appropriate, ask about personal needs and wishes. Assumptions are no alternative to seeking and respecting the wishes of individual patients. Good communications are central to effective, culturally sensitive healthcare. The healthcare professional must never discriminate against a patient for whatever reason, including cultural beliefs. Differences in cultural beliefs must be set aside, with the interests of the patient being put first and foremost.

Cultural Groups

This section summarises the basic characteristics of the main world cultures. It should be read against the background of the various religions (see Section 2). Cultures can sometimes be easily identified as a distinct group. Distinguishing cultures from countries can, however, be difficult. For example, Indians, of whom there are vast numbers in India, are also found in many countries worldwide. The same applies to Chinese. Distinguishing some cultures from religions can be impossible – for example, Judaism and Jews and Islam and Arabs. Since there is a large part of the world occupied by Arabs, and since most Arabs are Muslim and religious, we have included Arabs as a culture.

The section should be used as outlined in Table 3-1.

Africans

Africa is a very large continent that contains around 10% of the world population, with a heterogeneous but essentially Black African indigenous population living in many different countries, with sometimes vastly different climates, ethnic groups, cultures and religions. The knowledge base to be culturally sensitive to all the different peoples of Africa and those of African descent spread widely across the Americas and Europe is enormous. Countries of Africa can be grouped geographically, such as those in:

Table 3-1 **Information outlined in Section 3**

Contents	Details
Countries	Countries relevant to the culture
Population	Main population groups, relevant to ethnic background. Virtually all cultures also contain unrelated ethnic minorities
Religions (main)	Main religions and faiths, relevant to lifestyle and healthcare. Virtually all cultures also have religious minorities
Languages (main)	Main languages, relevant to communication. In virtually all cultures, the more educated individuals can communicate in English
Culture	Comments in addition to generalisations evident from the religious affiliations, such as family structure and behaviour
Greeting	Main points
Dietary and other habits and restrictions	General points about diet and habits such as alcohol and tobacco use
Health and healing traditions	Attitudes to HCPs, westernised and traditional medicine, restrictions and fears, time orientation
Oral health issues	Any salient points

- *North Africa, in which there are mainly Arabs and Berbers:* Algeria, Egypt (Arab Republic of), Libya (Great Socialist People's Libyan Arab Jamahiriya), Mauritania (Islamic Republic of), Morocco (Kingdom of), Tunisia (Tunisian Republic) and Western Sahara.
- *North East Africa, in which there are mainly Arabs:* Djibouti (Republic of), Eritrea (State of), Ethiopia (Federal Democratic Republic of), Somalia (including Somaliland) and Sudan (Republic of).

- *Islands, in which the population has largely a West African heritage:* of Cape Verde (West Africa), Comoros (Union of the), Madagascar, Mauritius (Republic of), São Tomé and Príncipe (Democratic Republic of) and Seychelles.
- Sub-Saharan Africa, which consists primarily of people of black African descent:
  - Central Africa: Angola, Cameroon, Central African Republic, Chad (Republic of), Democratic Republic of the Congo (formerly Zaire), Equatorial Guinea (Republic of), Gabon (Gabonese Republic), and Zambia
  - East Africa: Burundi (Republic of Burundi (formerly Urundi)), Kenya, Mozambique, Rwanda, Tanzania, Uganda
  - Southern Africa: Botswana, Congo (Republic of), Lesotho (Kingdom of), Malawi, Namibia, South Africa, Swaziland, and Zimbabwe
  - West Africa: Benin (Republic of), Burkina Faso, Côte d'Ivoire, Gambia (Republic of), Ghana, Guinea, Guinea-Bissau, Liberia, Mali, Niger, Nigeria, Senegal, Sierra Leone, and Togo.

History

The indigenous population of Africa is essentially Black African, but it has been colonised by Europeans over the centuries (Italians [Romans], Greeks, British, French, Belgians, Germans, Portuguese, Spanish, Dutch). African immigrants from the colonies are found in these European countries, and European descendants are to be found in many of the former African colonies. These are mainly:

- French in Algeria and other areas of North and West Africa in particular, including what are now Tunisia, Madagascar, Mauritania, Mali, Niger, Chad, Central African Republic, Congo, Gabon, Burkina faso, Cote d'Ivoire, Guinea, Senegal and Benin;
- Italians in what are now Eritrea, Libya and Ethiopia;
- Germans in Rwanda, Burundi, Tanzania, Togo and Namibia;
- Spanish in Equatorial Guinea, Morocco and the Western Sahara;
- Portuguese in Angola, Mozambique and Guinea-Bissau;
- Belgians to the Democratic Republic of the Congo;
- British in Egypt, Libya, Sudan, Ethiopia, Uganda, Zimbabwe, Zambia, Malawi, Botswana, Gambia, Ghana, Nigeria and Kenya;
- British, French, Germans and Dutch in South Africa. The descendants of the latter, the Afrikaners, are the largest white group in South Africa.
- Asians, particularly from the Indian subcontinent, came to the former British colonies of South Africa, Kenya and Uganda and neighbouring countries such as Tanzania. Thus English is widely spoken throughout Africa (Fig 3-1).

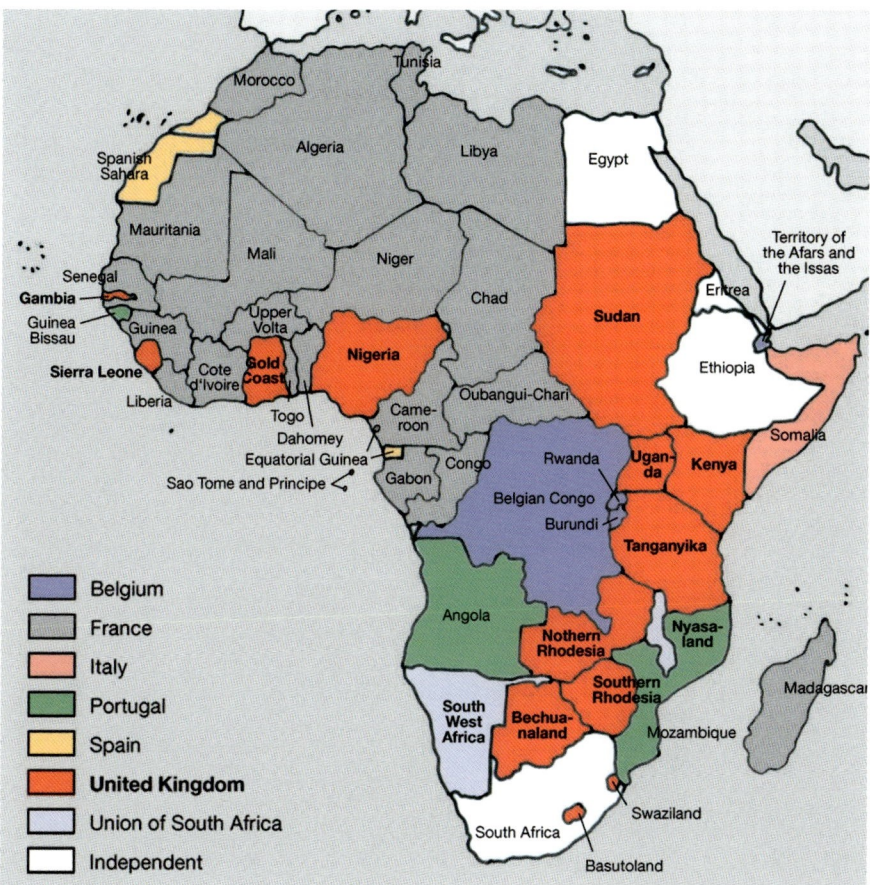

Fig 3-1 European influence in Africa.

- Also, having close proximity to the Middle East, there is a strong Arabic influence in the north and east of Africa and a significant Lebanese presence in West and Southern Africa.

Years of slavery, in which West Africans in particular were dispatched to the Americas at the hands of Europeans, Arabs and black Africans, resulted in the many diverse people of Africa being widely distributed throughout the world (Fig 3-2), living in either fully integrated or multicultural societies, mainly in the south of USA, the Caribbean and Central America, and the north of South America, as well as in the former imperialist countries and countries geographically close to Africa.

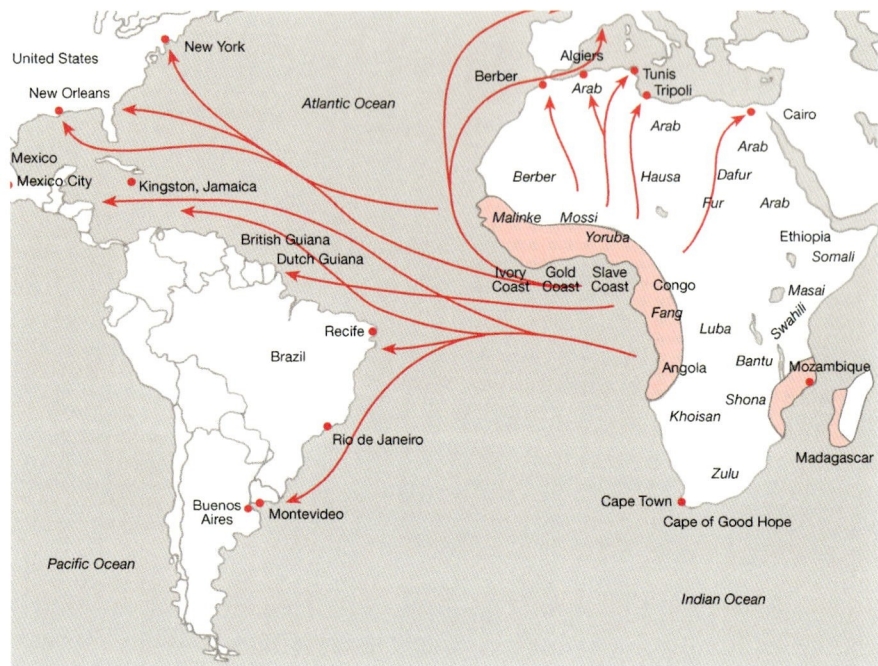

Fig 3-2 Migration of peoples from Africa.

Population

Black Africans predominate especially in West and sub-Saharan Africa, and are largely of Bantu origin. There is, however, a wide variety of physical types of black Africans from the tall Masai to Pygmies (of whom there are various tribes - Mbuti; Efe; Sua; Twa) who are among the world's shortest adults. Arabic speaking Arab-Berber Africans predominate in North and parts of North-Eastern Africa. Some Ethiopian/Eritrean groups (like the Amhara and Tigray -or 'Habesha') have semitic/Middle Eastern (Sabaen) ancestry. Most Somali clans also have Arab ancestry (although many of the 'Arabs' of Sudan clearly have African ancestry and are far off in appearance to Arabs in, for example, Yemen or Iran), but ethnic Somalis originated in the Ethiopian highlands. The significant differences in the populations in Africa between North Africa and sub-Saharan Africa is very obvious in countries such as Sudan and Mauritania, which are divided between a mostly Arab north and a black African south.

Peoples and ethnic/social groups include Afar, Anlo Ewe, Amhara, Arabic, Ashanti, Bakongo, Bambara, Bemba, Berber, Bobo, Bushmen/San, Chewa, Dogon, Fang, Fon, Fulani, Ibos, Kikuyu (Gikuyu) , Maasai, Mandinka, Pygmies, Samburu, Senufo, Tuareg, Wolof, Yoruba and Zulu.

Religions
Approximately 40% of all Africans are Christians (mainly in sub-Saharan Africa) and another 40% Muslims, who form the majority of the population north of the Sahara, and significant minorities in some sub-Saharan countries such as Nigeria and Kenya.

Roughly 20% of Africans primarily follow indigenous African religions that revolve around animism (the belief that personalised supernatural beings [or souls] inhabit all objects and govern their existence) and ancestor worship. A common thread is the division of the spiritual world into helpful spirits, which include ancestor spirits that help their descendants and protect communities from natural disaster or attacks, and harmful spirits, which include the souls of murdered victims who were buried without the proper funeral rites and spirits used by hostile spirit mediums to cause illness in their enemies. A minority of Africans have Judaic-based beliefs, such as the Beta Israel and Lemba.

Languages
Over a thousand languages are spoken in Africa, as well as European languages – especially English, French, Portuguese and Spanish. The four major vernacular language families (Table 3-2) are:
• Niger-Congo – probably the largest language family in the world, but most are Bantu languages, and spoken in sub-Saharan Africa.
• Afro-Asiatic – about 240 languages, widespread throughout North and East Africa, the Sahel (the area of central Africa just south of the Sahara), and Southwest Asia.
• Nilo-Saharan – more than 100 languages, spoken mainly in Chad, Sudan, Ethiopia, Uganda, Kenya, and northern Tanzania.
• Khoisan – about 50 languages, spoken mainly in Southern Africa.

English and French are the official languages of a significant portion of the African population, an outcome of colonisation.

Culture
Africans are generally friendly, gracious and hospitable. They are socially warm people, often touching and hugging, even between members of the same sex. They are modest and respectful, and often religious. Attitude towards

125

time may be flexible, and work/life balance may favour quality of life. Non-verbal gestures are common and there is often an oral culture, involving proverbs, jokes and stories.

Family structure varies considerably, but a nuclear family is common, often including widowed parents and single, female parents. Families tend to be matriarchal. Friends are often included in the support system. The father is typically the leader, provider, decision-maker and spokesman; the wife is the carer. However, the latter may increasingly be involved in decision-making. In some groups, the wife, once the husband dies, has to be 'cleansed' by a male relative having sexual intercourse with her – a tradition (kulowakufa) that may contribute to the transmission of HIV. There is a strong tradition of mutual support and respect for elders. Children are expected to be polite to, and respectful of, their elders who, in turn, often help raise the children.

Once older people lose their independence, they are typically housed with, and cared for by, their oldest child. Institutionalisation of older people and those with disability is not encouraged. If hospitalised, Africans tend to be cared for by family members who take turns at the bedside.

Greetings
see Section 2

Dietary and Other Habits and Restrictions
The food and drink of Africa reflect local and colonial influences, but is a combination of traditional fruits and vegetables, milk and meat products. Traditional African cuisine is characterised by use of starch as a focus, accompanied by stew containing meat or vegetables, or both. Cassava and yams are the main root vegetables. Africans also use steamed greens with hot spices. The African village diet is often milk, curds and whey. Watermelon, banana and plantain are some of the more familiar fruits.

The most familiar alcoholic drink in interior Africa is the Ethiopian honey wine called Tej.

Health and Healing Traditions
Africa is a continent where, despite the exploitation of oil and mineral resources, the per capita income is still very low, and a significant proportion of countries are developing nations. The population is largely young, and is rapidly increasing in most countries, but life expectation is predictably lower than in westernised societies, often by 20 or more years and increas-

ingly so given civil conflict, the spread of HIV/AIDS, and falling levels of state expenditure on health and social services. Tribal warfare is common, in particular in sub-Saharan Africa, with a number of instances of genocides. Drought, locusts, conflicts and other factors mean that malnutrition is common. This predisposes, along with climatic conditions, inadequate clean water and hygiene, to various communicable infections.

Throughout Africa, viruses, bacteria, or parasites can contaminate food or water and may cause diarrhoea and vomiting (*E. coli*, salmonella, cholera and parasites), fever (typhoid fever and toxoplasmosis) or liver damage (hepatitis). Viral hepatitis is endemic, as is tuberculosis (TB). Whooping cough, syphilis and gonorrhea common. Over the past decade the number of people with TB has tripled. TB is the leading killer of people with AIDS in Africa and the two form a lethal co-epidemic. Most African countries with high rates of TB are losing ground against the infectious disease.

Schistosomiasis (Bilharziasis), and guinea worm are parasitic infections found in fresh water. Schistosomiasis – caused by blood flukes that use freshwater snails as an intermediate host and invade humans when the larvae penetrate the skin of people entering a pond, lake, or stream in which the snails live – results in chronic debilitation. Guinea worm is a parasite spread through ingestion of contaminated water, endemic especially in many rural areas of sub-Saharan Africa, causing recurring illness. Onchocerciasis (river blindness) – caused by filarial worms transmitted by black flies that live and breed near rapidly flowing water – can damage the eyes and optic nerve and cause blindness. Malaria and yellow fever are endemic in many areas. Dengue, filariasis and leishmaniasis are other insect-borne diseases that occur in Africa. In North Africa there is a limited risk of malaria in parts of Algeria, Egypt and Morocco, but no risk of yellow fever. In Southern Africa there is a risk from malaria but not yellow fever. African tick bite fever, a rickettsial infection, is common in South Africa, Botswana, Swaziland, Lesotho and Zimbabwe. African sleeping sickness (African trypanosomiasis), which is transmitted through the bite of an infected tsetse fly, can occur in Botswana and Namibia. In East, Central and West Africa there is a risk from malaria, yellow fever, African sleeping sickness and rickettsial infections.

HIV appears to have originated in the area of the Congo or Cameroon and is ravaging much of sub-Saharan Africa where at least 10%, and in some areas up to 40%, of the population are infected and, until recently, had no access to anti-retroviral medications. By 2005, an estimated 25 million Africans had HIV infection and 16 million had died from AIDS. Indeed, 60% of the world's AIDS sufferers live in Africa.

Other lethal viral infections such as hepatitis viruses, Ebola virus and Lassa fever are also endemic, and outbreaks of meningitis, measles and other infections are common. Polio is still endemic in Nigeria.

African cultures may view health and disease and healthcare in a strikingly different fashion from Anglo-Americans. Indeed, entire systems of healing are built upon indigenous beliefs and traditions, and patients may hold very different understandings of health and disease.

Involvement with people and completion of interpersonal encounters is more valued than 'being on time'. The patient may expect the HCP to have all the answers and make all the decisions. Patients may regard as sensitive issues, matters that are sometimes more freely discussed by westernised patients. Head-nodding and smiles do not always signify comprehension or agreement; some patients are reluctant openly to disagree with HCPs.

The patient may take a passive role, answering but not asking questions, and waiting for the HCP to impart their diagnosis and recommendations. Most of the time medical or dental advice is accepted without question, but if the Western treatment fails to bring immediate relief of the symptoms, the patient may seek the care of a traditional physician or healer. The same thing may happen if a Western diagnosis is rejected because it bears a negative prognosis (including diagnosis of a long-term illness or of an illness that cannot be fully cured) or because surgery is advised. The traditional treatment may either replace the Western treatment or be used along with it. Many patients do not disclose the use of traditional care and medications to their Western HCPs because the two medical domains – Western and traditional medicine – are seen as entirely separate. Some patients may also fear that the Western HCP (an authority figure) will disapprove, or they believe that disclosure of the traditional care would violate the relationship of trust.

In terms of oral healthcare patients may hold very different understandings of health and disease. Some patients may, due to cultural or historical experiences, expect tooth conservation, but others may expect extraction. High prices or lack of access to treatment may lead to neglect of dental care where this is not seen as a priority.

Arabs

Terminology

* 'Arab' – the name originally applied to a Semitic person of the Arabian peninsula; now used also for a person who is a national of an Arab state, has command of the Arabic language, and possesses a fundamental knowledge of Arabian culture.
* 'Arabia' – the peninsula in South West Asia containing the world's largest known reserves of oil and natural gas. It is politically divided between Saudi Arabia (the largest and most populous nation), Yemen, Oman, the United Arab Emirates, Qatar, Bahrain and Kuwait. Jordan and Iraq are to the north, the Red Sea to the west, and the Persian Gulf to the east.
* 'Middle East' – the region that includes South West Asia and part of North East Africa, which includes the Asian part of Turkey, Syria, Israel, Jordan, Iraq; Iran, Lebanon, the countries of the Arabian peninsula, Egypt and Libya. The region was the site of great ancient civilizations, e.g., Mesopotamia and Egypt, and the birthplace of Judaism, Christianity and Islam. It contains much of the world's oil reserves and has many strategic trade routes, e.g. the Suez Canal. In the 20/21st century the area has been the scene of political turmoil and major warfare, e.g. in various Imperialist incursions; World War I; World War II; the Arab-Israeli Wars; the Iran-Iraq War and the (Persian) Gulf Wars.

Arab countries

Arabs are found especially in the Middle East. However, Afghanistan, Mauritania, Somalia, Sudan and Zanzibar also have large Arab populations.

History

A significant proportion of Arab countries are developed nations not least because the successful exploitation of oil and mineral resources has given a high per capita income, resulting in large numbers of guest workers, especially from South and South-East Asia. In contrast, some Arabs have moved to other countries because of political tensions and conflicts, or for employment, and for issues pertaining to quality of life.

Religion

Islam is by far the predominant religion, with religious beliefs and observance tending to be strong.

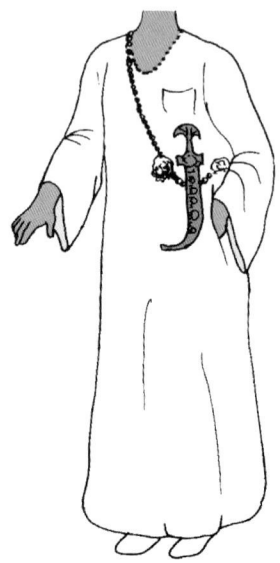

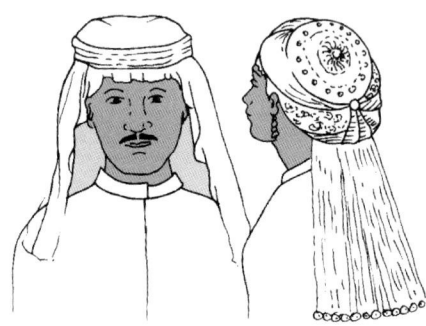

Fig 3-3 Dishdash.   **Fig 3-4** Keffiyehs.

Languages

Arabic is the language of the Qur`an, and the religious language of all Muslims and most Arabs. Many Arabs may also be fluent in English or French.

Culture

Arabs tend to be very polite, respectful, and often religious and proud. They dislike outward disagreements, and this can lead to responses that they believe others want. Thus neither head-nodding nor smiles can be taken always to mean either comprehension or agreement.

An extended family is common, often including widowed parents. Families tend to be matriarchal; the father is the leader, provider, and spokesman; the wife is the carer, but the grandmother and wife may be involved in decision-making. There is a strong tradition of mutual support and respect for elders. In family life, elders are respected and children tend to be 'seen but not heard'. Children are sacred but expected to be obedient, polite to and respectful of their elders who, in turn, often help raise the children. Once older people lose their independence, they are typically housed with, and cared for by, their oldest child. Institutionalisation of older people or those with disability is not encouraged.

If hospitalised, Arabs tend to be cared for by family members who take turns at the bedside, and failure so to do may be interpreted as lack of caring.

Traditional Arab dress for men is a tunic (dishdash) and headscarf (keffiyeh) (Figs 3-3 and 3-4).

Greetings

In addressing Arabs, the use of the appropriate title before the name is appropriate. Women rarely change their name when they marry. In the Middle East, Arabs like using the title – e.g. Dr, Mr, Professor, or to be called Abu (father of) the name of the first born child, e.g. Abu Faisal (father of Faisal).

Dietary and Other Habits and Restrictions

Arabs are not permitted to eat pork or drink alcohol. Food, especially meat, must be Halal. Seafood of most kinds is permitted. Many Arabs away from home may limit themselves to a vegetarian diet.

Health and Healing Traditions

The population is largely young, rapidly increasing in most Arab countries, and life expectation is about the same as in westernised societies.

Areas of Iran, Iraq, Oman, Saudi Arabia, the Syrian Arab Republic, Turkey and Yemen are a risk for malaria, but there is no risk for yellow fever in the Middle East, and HIV is only at a low prevalence. Viruses, bacteria or parasites, which are found throughout the Middle East, can contaminate food or water and may cause diarrhoea and vomiting (*E. coli*, salmonella, cholera, and parasites), fever (typhoid fever and toxoplasmosis) or liver damage (hepatitis). Cutaneous leishmaniasis is reported throughout the region and visceral leishmaniasis is common in central Iraq, in south west Saudi Arabia, in the north west of Syria, in Turkey (south east Anatolia), and in west Yemen. A rise in West Nile fever has been seen recently in Israel. Outbreaks of dengue occur in Saudi Arabia and Yemen. Other infections in this region include tuberculosis (Yemen), lymphatic filariasis and onchocerciasis (Yemen), hepatitis B, and schistosomiasis (Saudi Arabia, Yemen, Iraq and Syria), and Polio has resurfaced in Yemen. Pilgrims to the Hajj in Saudi Arabia have acquired meningococcal infections caused by serotypes A and W-135, as well as influenza.

Anglo-American healthcare values are often adopted, characterised by beliefs in individualism, informed consent, science and technology, orientation towards clock time and separation of health from spiritual health significantly affect healthcare. Disease may be thought to be caused by bad luck, stress and unfavourable environments, and the 'evil eye'. Many Arabs may wear an amulet to ward off the 'evil eye'.

Whilst it is impossible to generalise, the people are not always time-oriented, modesty is valued, especially by women, and expectations of HCPs may be high.
Involvement with people and completion of interpersonal encounters is more valued than 'being on time'. Family members often accompany the patient for appointments, and their involvement in decision-making is typical, with the father or eldest son being the spokesperson.

In issues of consent, great store is placed in trust. The concept of written consent may prove difficult, as agreements are often made in good faith alone. Treatment should be avoided on Fridays and during Ramadan, unless after sunset, when drugs, if needed, are best prescribed once a day, again after sunset. There may be non-compliance with oral medication regimes during fasts such as Ramadan.

Oral Healthcare Issues
Arab acceptance of routine dental care is often high; however, there may be simultaneous home care of certain conditions, involving traditional remedies. The use of local and general anaesthetic and sedation should not be an issue, subject to clear explanation and justification of the need to use such techniques.

Agents and oral health products free of alcohol and animal products such as gelatin should be selected wherever possible.

Australasians

Countries
Australasia is a term referring to Australia and New Zealand and their external territories. Oceania in wider use includes Australia but is sometimes used more narrowly as a term for varying groups of islands of the Pacific Ocean viz:
- Melanesia (Fiji – Republic; New Caledonia - collectivity of France; Papua New Guinea - Commonwealth Realm; Solomon Islands - Commonwealth Realm; and Vanuatu - Republic);
- Micronesia (Guam – organized, unincorporated territory of the United States; Kiribati - Republic; Marshall Islands - Republic in free association with the USA; Micronesia, Federated States of - Republic in free association with the United States; Nauru - Republic; Northern Mariana Islands

- organised, unincorporated commonwealth in political union with the United States; Palau - Republic in free association with the United States; Wake - unorganised, unincorporated territory of the United States); and

• Polynesia (American Samoa – unorganised, unincorporated territory of the United States; Cook Islands - self-governing state in free association with New Zealand; French Polynesia - 'overseas country' of France; Nike - self-governing state in free association with New Zealand; New Zealand - Commonwealth Realm; Pitcairn - overseas territory of the United Kingdom; Samoa - constitutional monarchy under Malietoa Tanumafili II;Tokelau - semi-autonomous territory of Zealand; Tonga - absolute monarchy under King Taufa'ahau Tupou IV; Tuvalu - Commonwealth Realm; Wallis - overseas collectivity of France).

History

Britain has influenced the culture of Australasia from former colonisation when the indigenous populations, the Australian aboriginals and the New Zealand Maoris were subjugated for centuries. Immigration was encouraged from Britain and Europe, and occurred from South East Asia and the Pacific Rim, following the Korean, Vietnamese and other wars in the 1950s and 1970s.

Population

Most of the Australasian population originates from UK, as well as minorities largely from Europe and South East Asia.

Religions

Mainly Christianity.

Languages

Mainly English.

Culture

Australasia has a westernised culture and lifestyle. Whilst it is impossible to generalise, the people are often conscious of the need for punctuality. However, as in most other parts of the world, society, culture and lifestyles are changing in Australasia. A feature of this change is increasing homogeneity; however, national characteristics are anticipated to remain apparent for the foreseeable future. For example, English is used in communications, notably in electronic media, including the internet.

Dietary and Other Habits and Restrictions

The dietary and other habits and restrictions of Australasians, while still tend-

133

ing to reflect national customs and cuisines of the various immigrant groups, are very mixed. Overall the diet of Australasians, despite health promotion campaigns, may be found to be conducive to conditions including cardio-vascular disease, diabetes and obesity, with many diets being cariogenic. Smoking and alcohol use remains prevalent in Australasia, in particular in lower socioeconomic groups and young adults across the social spectrum.

Health and Healing Traditions

Australia and New Zealand have most of the health issues of any developed nation. Viruses, bacteria, or parasites, which are found throughout Australia and the South Pacific, can contaminate food or water and may cause diar-rhoea and vomiting (*E. coli*, salmonella, cholera, and parasites), fever (typhoid fever and toxoplasmosis), or liver damage (hepatitis). In the region there are malaria-risk areas in Papua New Guinea, the Solomon Islands and Vanuatu. There is no risk for malaria in Australia, Christmas Island, Cook Island, Fed-erated States of Micronesia, Fiji, French Polynesia (Tahiti), Guam, Kiribati, Marshall Islands, Nauru, New Caledonia, New Zealand, Niue, Northern Mariana Islands, Palau, Pitcairn, Samoa, American Samoa, Tokelau, Tonga, Tuvalu, Wake Island, Wallis and Futuna. There is no yellow fever in this region. Dengue, filariasis, Ross River virus, and Murray Valley encephalitis are diseases carried by insects in this region. Scrub typhus and other rick-ettsial infections are present. Japanese encephalitis is present in Papua New Guinea and the Torres Strait and far northern Australia. Other hazards include ciguatera poisoning (from consumption of subtropical and tropical marine finfish that have accumulated naturally occurring dinoflagellate tox-ins through their diet), which occurs frequently on some of the islands, snake and spider bites. There are serious problems in some areas related to the acquisition, supply and use of drugs of dependence, and their social and health consequences, with blood-borne infections such as HIV and hepatitis viruses, crime and violence.

Anglo-American values are widespread, summarised by beliefs in individu-alism, informed consent, science and technology, orientation towards clock time and separation of health from spiritual health significantly affect health-care. Health and healthcare provision is a major concern of Australasians of all ages.

Oral Healthcare Issues

Water fluoridation is common although not universal throughout Australa-sia, with a beneficial effect on caries incidence in the fluoridated areas. Den-tal care is well accepted throughout Australasia. Attitudes and access to dental care may, however, be found to be very variable, with many Australasian, especially indigenous peoples, either not seeking routine dental care, or being unable to access or afford even basic oral healthcare provision. It is suggested that interest in oral health and, in particular, dental attractiveness is increasing, as evidenced by a steady growth in the range and sale of oral hygiene and related products.

As in many parts of the world, there are new emerging dental needs and demands amongst, for example, the elderly who are living longer and retaining more teeth throughout life.

Caribbeans (West Indians)

Countries
The Caribbean or the West Indies is a group of islands in the Caribbean Sea. They include:
* British West Indies/Anglophone Caribbean - Anguilla, Antigua and Barbuda, Bahamas, Barbados, British Virgin Islands, Cayman Islands, Dominica, Grenada, Jamaica, Montserrat, Saint Kitts and Nevis, Saint Lucia, Saint Vincent and the Grenadines, Trinidad and Tobago and the Turks and Caicos Islands. Guyana (formerly British Guiana) is included within the West Indians from a cultural perspective; although Guyana is on the South American mainland, it shares a common history with the peoples of the Caribbean.
* Danish West Indies - present-day United States Virgin Islands.
* Dutch West Indies - present-day Netherlands Antilles and Aruba; Suriname (formerly Dutch Guiana).
* French West Indies - Haiti and the French overseas départements of Guadeloupe, Martinique and French Guiana.
* Spain - Cuba, Hispaniola (present-day Dominican Republic and Haiti), and Puerto Rico.

History
Most islands were originally populated by indigenous people and at some point were – and a minority still are – colonies of European nations. The colonial leaders first took the indigenous people to work in mines and in agriculture. As many of the indigenous groups of the Caribbean died out under the extreme regimes, the owners of the mines and farms replaced them with forced labour from further afield. Today, the majority of people are of black African descent whose forefathers were brought across as slaves – many to work in sugar plantations; people of Indian descent – whose fore-

fathers were taken over as indentured labour as slavery declined; and people of Chinese descendent – many of whose forefathers were also indentured workers. Today, many Caribbeans have a mixed racial heritage.

Being close to the USA, European and American influences are strong. Many Caribbeans have emigrated to Europe and USA. At the time of the Second World War, the countries of the British Caribbean were still colonies and, on request, many men came to support the UK and fought for 'the mother country'. As prosperity and economic growth returned post-war in the 1950s, the UK actively recruited people in the Caribbean to come to the UK to work in public transport and the National Health Service. Many responded to this second call and came in search of work and improved living conditions. Europe and the USA continue to recruit skilled workers, particularly nurses, from the Caribbean.

Population
Due to their history, Caribbeans tend to be highly ethnically diverse, but a significant number may be able to trace at least part of their ancestry to West Africa or the Indian sub-continent.

Religions
The distribution of religious faiths mirrors colonial heritage and language. Therefore, among African descendants, Christianity is the majority religion, with Roman Catholicism the predominant faith in the French and Spanish speaking countries and Protestantism the norm in the former British, now Commonwealth, and Dutch Caribbean countries. Trinidad is one of the largest Caribbean islands where the proportion of people of African and Indian descent are similar. Two thirds of people are aligned with Christian-based religions, with around one third ascribed to Hinduism and Islam. Those following the Muslim faith (10%) have shown rapid growth in recent years.

Indigenous, or sycretic, faiths are common in some areas. Voodou originated in Haiti during the French colonial period and is still practised there. It is based on tribal religions of West Africa with influences from the indigenous Indian population. The slave owners forbade the practice of native religions and baptised all slaves as Catholics. Therefore, Catholicism became super-imposed and, since native religions were forbidden, voodou was practised covertly and may still be denied today. Catholic saints became absorbed into voodou, so that the presence of their pictures cannot necessarily be taken as representative of the practice of Christianity. Minority religions include Judaism, Islam, Hinduism, Bahá'ís and Rastafarianism.

Languages

Depending on their European heritage, languages include French, Spanish, Dutch, with English common across the region. Many Caribbean nations have their own African- influenced Creole versions of European languages with words and sounds originating from a combination of European stress accent languages and West African tonal languages. Language is generally English/Patois (Black English), or possibly French or Spanish.

Culture

Many stereotypes exist to describe West Indian people, and beliefs and behaviours reflect the major influences that formed the diversity of communities that exist today. During slavery, marriage between African people was often forbidden – a possible legacy in modern times being a history of the acceptance of single mothers in some social groups. Similarly, slaves were discouraged from looking at slave owners eye to eye. Generations of teaching children to look down has led to claims that black men may be perceived to be evasive when challenged by authority.

People from the Caribbean are typically friendly, gracious and hospitable. Touching between members of the same sex is common. Due to a migrant history with access to education initially controlled, a rich oral culture developed, involving proverbs, jokes and stories. Older generations may be modest and respectful, and often religious. Attitude towards time may be flexible, and work/life balance may favour quality of life. Involvement with people and completion of interpersonal encounters is more valued than 'being on time'. Family structure varies considerably, but a nuclear family is common, often including widowed parents and single, female parents. Families tend to be matriarchal, and friends are often included in the support system. In nuclear families, especially first-generation migrants, the father was typically the leader, provider, decision-maker and spokesman; the wife taking the lead caring role. In modern times, mothers often go ahead when families migrate, becoming the major wage earner, with money sent 'home'.

Within family networks, there is a strong tradition of mutual support and respect for elders. Children are expected to be polite to, and respectful of, their elders who, in turn, often help raise the children (Fig 3-5). Once older people lose their independence, they are typically housed with, and cared for by, their oldest child. Institutionalisation of older people or those with disability is not encouraged. If hospitalised, they tend to be cared for by family members who take turns at the bedside.

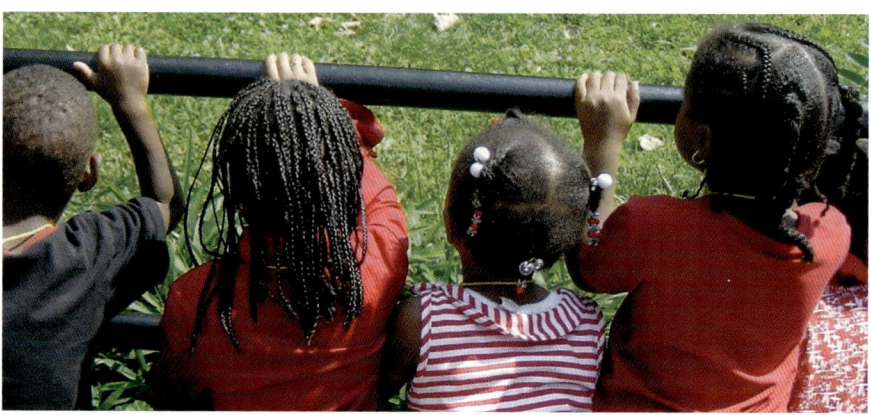

Fig 3-5 Children of a Caribbean family.

Dietary and Other Habits and Restrictions
Increasingly, the diet of Caribbeans may be formed to be a mixture of traditional and western foods and dishes.

Health and Healing Traditions
A significant proportion of the Carribean countries are developing nations. The population is rapidly increasing in most countries, but resources are scarce and the per capita income is generally low. Malaria is endemic, as are other parasitic infections. HIV is on the increase. There are serious problems in some areas related to the acquisition, supply and use of drugs of dependence, and their social and health consequences, with blood-borne infections such as HIV and hepatitis viruses, crime and violence.

Caribbean people may have a different view of the importance of time and punctuality to Anglo-Americans, although, if the importance of healthcare appointments is stressed, this is not necessarily a problem. Involvement with people and completion of interpersonal encounters is more valued than 'being on time'. Lunchtime and early afternoon 'siestas' are not uncommon, and are not always the best times to arrange appointments.

Same-gender HCPs may be preferred. It is not uncommon that nurses are expected to be female. Caribbean patients may have some difficulty understanding why consent should be written and signed. They are often private and modest people and may be most unhappy if their condition were to be

138

discussed with family or friends without their express consent. Interpreters may not be trusted if the patient does not believe they will convey the intended messages, and then family may be preferred over friends, in order to maintain confidentiality.

Adoption of preventive care may be limited. Stigma related to several health issues is common – for example, in relation to mental illness and HIV/AIDS – and this can lead to under-reporting or late presentation. Patients may have a fear of surgery. Self-diagnosis and self-treatment are not uncommon. Home remedies may be used extensively, possibly together with prescribed treatments. Some systems of healing are built upon indigenous beliefs and traditions and patients may hold very different understandings of health and disease. Herbal teas (bush teas) are commonly used.

The patient may expect the HCP to have all the answers and make all the decisions. As a result, the patient takes a passive role, answering but not asking questions, and waiting for the HCP to impart their diagnosis and recommendations. Most of the time medical or dental advice appears to be accepted without question, even though a minority may be acted upon. Patients may regard as sensitive issues matters that are sometimes more freely discussed by westernised patients. Head-nodding and smiles do not always signify comprehension or agreement; some patients are reluctant openly to disagree with HCPs.

In some social groups, if the Western treatment fails to bring immediate relief of the symptoms, the patient may seek the care of a traditional physician or healer. The same thing may happen if a Western diagnosis is rejected because it bears a negative prognosis (including diagnosis of a long-term illness or of an illness that cannot be fully cured) or because surgery is advised. The traditional treatment may either replace the Western treatment or be used along with it. Many patients do not disclose the use of traditional care and medications to their Western HCPs because the two medical domains – Western and traditional medicine – are seen as entirely separate. Some patients may also fear that the Western HCP (an authority figure) will disapprove, or they believe that disclosure of the traditional care would violate the relationship of trust.

Increasingly, many Carribeans are adopting Anglo-American values summarised by beliefs in individualism, informed consent, science and technology, orientation towards clock time and separation of health from spiritual health significantly affect healthcare.

Oral Healthcare Issues

In terms of oral healthcare patients may hold very different understandings of health and disease from Westerners. Some patients may, due to cultural or historical experiences, expect tooth conservation, but others may expect extraction. High prices or lack of access to treatment may lead to neglect of dental care where this is not seen as a priority. Dental care is generally accepted, but may only be sought when in pain or discomfort.

Central Asians

Countries

Central Asia includes Afghanistan, Mongolia and the Commonwealth of Independent States (CIS) (a confederation of former Soviet Republics [Armenia, Azerbaijan, Belarus, Georgia, Kazakhstan, Kyrgyzstan, Moldova, Russia, Tajikistan, Turkmenistan, Ukraine, and Uzbekistan]).

History

Following the collapse in 1991 of the Soviet Union (Union of Soviet Socialist Republics: USSR), the Commonwealth of Independent States (CIS) emerged to include 11 former Soviet Republics, leaving the Russian Federation as a separate entity. Inter-ethnic conflicts are on-going in some areas.

Population

The population is heterogeneous, mainly nationals of the various republics.

Religions

Several of the countries are largely Muslim, others Christian.

Languages

The languages of most inhabitants of the former Soviet Republics come from the Turkic language group. Turkmen, closely related to Turkish, is mainly spoken in Turkmenistan and into Afghanistan, Iran and Turkey. Kazakh, Kyrgyz and Tatar are related Turkic languages, spoken throughout Kazakhstan, Kyrgyzstan and Tajikistan, and into Afghanistan, Xinjiang and Qinghai. Uzbek and Uighur are spoken in Uzbekistan, Tajikistan and Xinjiang.

Arabic is a common language across the region. Russian, as well as being spoken by the ethnic Russians of Central Asia, is a lingua franca throughout the former Soviet Central Asian Republics. Russian is considered an official language in Russia, Belarus, Kazakhstan and Kyrgyzstan and separatist regions of Abkhazia and Transnistria, as well as the semi-autonomous region of Gagauzia in Moldova. Chinese has an equally dominant presence in Nei Monggol, Qinghai and Xinjiang.

Culture
see Islam and Christianity.

Dietary and Other Habits and Restrictions
see Islam and Christianity.

Health and Healing Traditions
A significant proportion of the countries of Central Asia are developing nations. The early years of independence from the Soviet Union had a disastrous effect on public health, with a move away from universally available free healthcare. Furthermore, because of low pay, many HCPs have moved away. The population is rapidly increasing but resources are scarce and, despite the exploitation of oil and mineral resources, the per capita income is still very low. The population is largely young. Life expectation is lower than in westernised societies, often by 10 or more years.

Malnutrition and inter-ethnic conflict has been common, with a number of instances of genocide. There are serious problems in some areas related to the acquisition, supply and use of drugs of dependence, and their social and health consequences, with blood-borne infections such as HIV and hepatitis viruses, TB, crime and violence. Parts of Armenia, Azerbaijan, Georgia, Kyrgyzstan, Tajikistan, Turkmenistan and Uzbekistan have a malaria risk. Viruses, bacteria or parasites found throughout the region can contaminate food and water and may cause diarrhoea and vomiting (E. coli, salmonella, cholera, and parasites), fever (typhoid fever and toxoplasmosis), or liver damage (hepatitis). The risk of hepatitis A can be high in parts of the region. Other infections include hepatitis B, hepatitis C, rickettsial infections, encephalitis and, in parts of Azerbaijan and Tajikistan, cutaneous and visceral leishmaniasis.

Systems of healing are built upon indigenous beliefs and traditions, with patients holding very different understandings of health and disease from Anglo-Americans. Involvement with people and completion of interpersonal encounters is more valued than 'being on time'. The patient may expect the HCP to have all the answers and make all the decisions. As a result, the patient often takes a passive role, answering but not asking questions, and waiting for the HCP to impart their diagnosis and recommendations. Most of the time HCP advice is accepted without question.

Patients may regard as sensitive issues matters that are sometimes more freely discussed by westernised patients. Head-nodding and smiles do not always signify comprehension or agreement; some patients are reluctant openly to disagree with HCPs.

If the Western treatment fails to bring immediate relief of the symptoms, the patient may seek the care of a traditional physician or healer. The same thing may happen if a Western diagnosis is rejected because it bears a negative prognosis (including diagnosis of a long-term illness or of an illness that cannot be fully cured) or because surgery is advised. The traditional treatment may either replace the Western treatment or be used along with it. Many patients do not disclose the use of traditional care and medications to their Western HCPs because the two medical domains are seen as separate. Some patients may fear that the Western HCP (an authority figure) will disapprove, with disclosure of the traditional care violating the relationship of trust.

Oral Healthcare Issues (see Islam)
In terms of oral healthcare, patients may hold very different understandings of health and disease to those in the West. Some patients may, due to cultural or historical experiences, expect tooth conservation but others may expect extraction. High prices or lack of access to treatment may lead to neglect of dental care where this is not seen as a priority.

Chinese

Countries
People of Chinese heritage are found mainly in The People's Republic of China (PRC), but Chinese live in most parts of the world (Fig 3-6), especially in South East Asia, Canada, USA, and around the whole Pacific rim. They originate largely from mainland China, Taiwan, Hong Kong, Korea, Philippines, South East Asia or the South Pacific. The Chinese population is rapidly increasing in many countries and is generally young (Fig 3-7).

History
China is one of the few remaining communist countries but has established itself as a world economic power and is increasingly recognised as a global strategic power. Taiwan remains an independent republic but is claimed by the PRC to be part of China.

Population
PRC has a majority Han Chinese population (93%), but there are 56 recog-

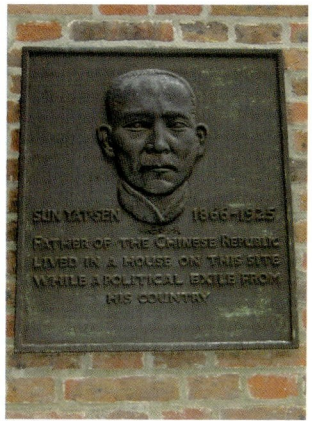

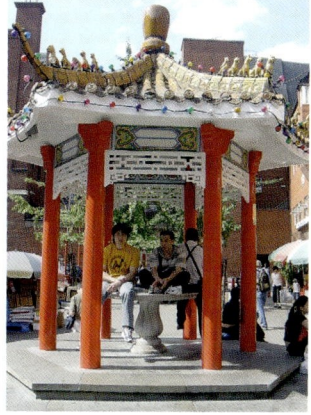

Fig 3-6 Plaque commemorating Sun Yat Sen, Chinese exil to the UK.

Fig 3-7 Young Chinese in China town, London.

nised ethnicities. Britain has influenced the culture of Hong Kong from former colonisation, but this has now been assimilated into China. Portugal influenced Macao.

Religions
Although mainly atheist, many Chinese are strongly influenced by Confucianism, Buddhism or Taoism. Chinese living arround the world may have adopted Western religions (Fig 3-8).

Festivals
- Yuan Tan (Chinese New Year); the first day of the first lunar month.
- Teng Chieh (Lantern Festival); the first full moon each year.

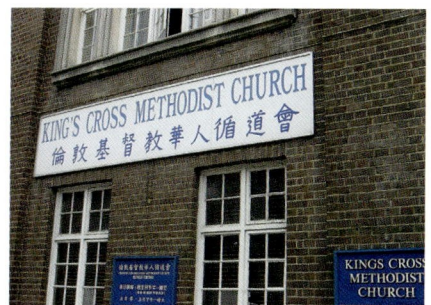

Fig 3-8 Chinese as part of acculturation may adopt other faiths.

143

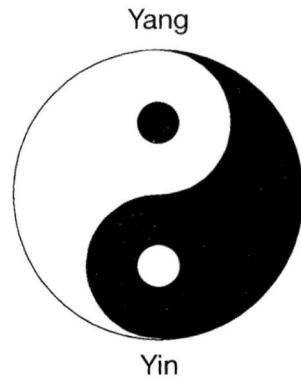

Yang

Yin   **Fig 3-9** Yin and Yang.

Languages
The majority of Chinese speak varieties of spoken Chinese, mainly Mandarin Chinese.

Culture
Despite diversity in culture, language, etiquette and social interactions, there are many cultural commonalities, especially amongst the older people of Chinese ancestry. Much is based on three schools of thought:
• Buddhism
• Confucianism
• Taoism.

Chinese people are typically gracious, hospitable and respectful. Loyalty, kindness, honour, reputation and harmony tend to be valued. They often have concerns about reputation and disagreements. Emotions are frowned upon. Chinese may hide personal feelings and be reluctant to question decisions and can appear abrupt. Gifts are commonly given, and older Chinese people are often keen to be charitable.

Yin and yang influence almost every aspect of the Chinese persons' view of the world: Yin represents the negative, dark, cold, feminine side of all things, and Yang represents the positive, bright, warm, masculine side of all things. Yin and yang must remain in balance and harmony (Fig 3-9). Good luck articles may be worn, such as jade or a rope around the waist.

Families are extended and patriarchal. The father is the leader, provider, decision-maker and spokesman; the wife is the carer. Traditional values persist amongst Chinese with respect to parents, elders and authority. Children are expected to be obedient, and polite to, and respectful of, their elders who, in turn, often help raise the children. There is a strong tradition of mutual support and respect for elders. Older people are typically housed with, and cared for by, their family. Institutionalisation of older people and those with disability is not encouraged. If hospitalised, they tend to be cared for by family members who take turns at the bedside. Failure so to do may be interpreted as lack of caring.

In the Chinese naming system, the family name comes first, followed by a two-part personal name e.g. Leung Mee-Ling. The first part of the personal name may be shared by children. Women on marriage usually add the husband's family name before their own.

Eye contact is often avoided with 'superiors' as a mark of respect. Sitting with the legs crossed, or leaning on a table or desk, or pointing at anything with the foot when talking are considered signs of contempt toward the person being addressed. Use both hands to offer something.

Dietary and Other Habits and Restrictions
Many Chinese believe that Yin and Yang should be balanced in the diet, Yin ('cold') foods including, for example, fruit and vegetables, and Yan ('hot') foods including meat, eggs and fried foods.

Diet plays a major role in the Chinese way of life, with many preventive health measures and cures depending on regulating or changing the diet. Rice soup and chicken may be viewed as 'illness food' believed to diminish scar formation. Beef and eggs may not be served to those who are ill. Most Chinese are lactose-intolerant.

Most Chinese relish crunchy foods and like chewing cartilage and bone, resulting in heavy loading and possible failure of restored teeth. Many Chinese men smoke heavily and drink beer and rice wine.

Health and Healing Traditions
Despite China emerging from being a developing nation and now being a global power, there are several serious public health problems related especially to health, tobacco smoking, air and water pollution, and infectious diseases. HIV-AIDS is epidemic, hepatitis viruses are endemic and recent problems include TB, severe acute respiratory syndrome (SARS) , H5N1 avian flu, and *Streptococcus suis* infections. There is no risk for yellow fever, and malaria is rare apart

145

from some remote areas. Dengue, filariasis, Japanese encephalitis, leishmaniasis and plague are diseases carried by insects in this region. Viruses, bacteria or parasites, throughout China, can contaminate food or water and may cause diarrhoea and vomiting (*E. coli*, salmonella, cholera, and parasites), fever (typhoid fever and toxoplasmosis) or liver damage (hepatitis).

Chinese people will generally keep appointments on time, but do not like to take time off work. Modesty and privacy is very important, especially for Chinese women.

Gentle touch is appropriate, but not to head or feet; as most Chinese consider the head the most sacred part of the body. It should never be touched without first obtaining the patient's permission. Patients may regard as sensitive issues matters that are sometimes more freely discussed by Western patients. Head-nodding and smiles do not always signify comprehension or agreement; some patients are reluctant openly to disagree with HCPs. As Chinese people may be reluctant to question the views of healthcare professionals, securing informed consent may be problematical.

The patient may expect the HCP to have all the answers and make all the decisions. As a result, the patient takes a passive role, answering but not asking questions, and waiting for the HCP to impart their diagnosis and recommendations. Most of the time medical and dental advice is accepted without question.

Since everything that is Yin has a small amount of Yang in it, and vice versa, Chinese people tend to view things more in shades of grey rather than as absolutes. This sometimes makes it difficult for them to accept a Western diagnosis of a single 'cause' of a complaint or to rely on a single form of medical treatment or cure. Chinese patients tend to believe that injected medication is more effective than oral drugs but, in contrast, dislike venepuncture, which is regarded as weakening the body. Chinese patients may also be found to be unused to taking pills, preferring to take medicine in the form of a tea or a slurry. Chinese patients may reduce drug dosages since they often consider Western medicines 'hot' and too potent – especially to Chinese, who tend to be smaller in stature than most Westerners. The patient may even discontinue the medication completely without consulting the HCP if the symptoms abate or if there has been no relief of the symptoms within a few days. This, together with the strong belief in traditional Chinese medicine (TCM), the use of which may not be disclosed to Western healthcare professionals, may complicate some treatments.

146

Chinese patients may appear to understand a diagnosis and accept a treatment, but may still fail to comply. This may be attributable to the concepts of harmony and 'face'. To maintain both their own 'face' and the HCP's, patients may not admit that they do not understand the diagnosis or treatment plan, or will pretend to accept it when they disagree. Because of a cultural respect for harmony, patients who fail to understand a treatment or even disagree with it, may avoid disrupting harmony or causing conflict and suppress negative thoughts and emotions.

Therefore, HCPs should learn to observe the indirect (often nonverbal) communication signs that indicate confusion or displeasure, and should 'test' the patient's comprehension by asking the patient to describe what they have been told in their own words. Not surprisingly, doctor-shopping is common.

Very traditional Chinese (mainly those from mainland China and the older generation from Hong Kong or Singapore) are unwilling to agree to removal of any body part or to organ donation. This can affect a Chinese patient's attitude to surgery.

HCPs are often surprised when Chinese patients present them with a gift to enhance face. It is expected that a gift will be repaid by effective healthcare.

Many older immigrant Chinese may be lonely, unable or unwilling to travel, and are poor users of social services.

The entire Chinese system of healing is built upon indigenous beliefs and traditions. Patients may hold very different understandings of health and disease from those with Anglo-American values. If the Western treatment fails to bring immediate relief of the symptoms, the patient may seek the care of a traditional physician or healer. The same thing may happen if a Western diagnosis is rejected because it bears a negative prognosis (including diagnosis of a long-term illness or of an illness that cannot be fully cured) or involving surgery. The traditional treatment may either replace the Western treatment or be used along with it. Many patients do not disclose the use of traditional care and medications to their Western HCPs because the two medical domains – Western and traditional medicine – are seen as entirely separate. Some patients may fear that the Western HCP (an authority figure) will disapprove, or they believe that disclosure of the traditional care would violate the relationship of trust.

Traditional Chinese Medicine (TCM)

Most TCM is increasingly popular. TCM investigation involves a search for imbalances within the patient's physical and mental self (Fig 3-10). TCM treatment focuses on the restoration of balance, and includes acupuncture, herbs, soups, ginseng and various other natural products.

Everything in the universe is classified as either Yin, which is 'cold', or Yang, which is 'hot'. The terms refer not to temperatures, but to attributes and conditions based upon Yin and Yang. The hot/cold classification, which is applied as much to recently discovered diseases and biomedical treatments as to traditional ones, includes parts of the body and their functions, diseases, and medicines. A 'hot' disease is treated by a 'cold' medicine in order to rebalance the patient's condition. Linden tea, for example, which may be served hot, is considered a 'cold' herb and is used to treat 'hot' ailments. Penicillin, on the other hand, is considered a 'hot' treatment because it can produce diarrhoea and rashes, which are viewed as 'hot' symptoms. While not every Chinese patient subscribes to the traditional beliefs, no HCP can afford to ignore the possibility that a particular patient may be influenced by them to some degree. For example, water and fruit juice are 'cold' substances that are to be avoided during illness that produces a 'cold' condition. Consequently, Chinese patients may greatly curtail their fluid intake, since water conducts 'cold' into the body. If a Western-trained HCP prescribes cold fluids to a person with pyrexia, not only might the patient ignore the advice, but they might also question the expertise of the HCP.

TCM traditional treatments that leave welts difficult to distinguish from the bruises left by beatings, and which have been the source of misunderstanding between Chinese parents and western HCPs, include:

- Coining and pinching; a heated metal coin is rubbed briskly over the skin until welts appear. Similar welts can also be produced by pinching the skin between the thumb and index finger.
- Cupping; heating and applying small hot cups to the forehead or abdomen produce a negative pressure as they cool, causing a circular ecchymosis.
- Moxibustion; pulverised wormwood or other burning incense is applied to the torso, head, or neck to produce superficial burns.

Oral Healthcare Issues

In terms of oral healthcare patients may hold very different understandings of health and disease to Anglo-Americans. Most Chinese accept modern oral healthcare, but can be dubious and may prefer to attend a Chinese dentist who understands traditional Chinese medicine. There is often a belief in suscepti-

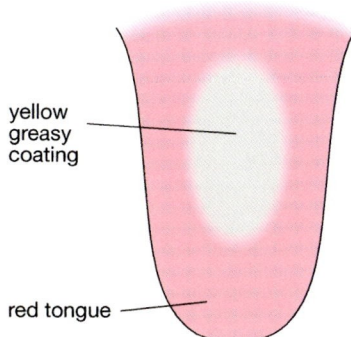

yellow
greasy
coating

red tongue

Fig 3-10 In traditional Chinese medicine an atypical appearance of the tongue, including coatings and redness is an indication of physical imbalance.

bility to dental disease, an expectation to loose teeth in old age, and a poor understanding of oral health issues. Dental care may rank low in patients' healthcare priorities, oral healthcare may be limited and attendance may be in the event of active problems only. Some patients may, due to cultural or historical experiences, expect tooth conservation but others may expect extraction. High prices or lack of access to treatment may lead to neglect of dental care where this is not seen as a priority.

Healthcare professionals, including dentists, tend to be held in high regard, but are expected to demonstrate competence and professionalism.

East Asians

(see Chinese)

Europeans

Countries
The European Union (EU) is a union of 25 independent states based on the European Communities and founded to enhance political, economic and social cooperation. It was formerly known as the European Community (EC) or European Economic Community (EEC). At the beginning of 2006, the 25 members were Austria, Belgium, Denmark, Finland, France, Germany, Greece, Ireland, Italy, Luxembourg, Netherlands, Portugal, Spain, Sweden, United Kingdom of Great Britain and Northern Ireland, Cyprus (Greek part), the Czech Republic, Estonia, Hungary, Latvia, Lithuania, Malta, Poland, Slovakia and Slovenia. In 2005, negotiations began to consider

including Turkey and Croatia. Albania, Bosnia and Herzegovina, Bulgaria, Iceland, Macedonia, Moldova, Norway, Romania, Serbia and Montenegro and Switzerland.

History

Europe has a diverse culture, arising from a long and turbulent history with numerous wars and invasions, population migrations and political changes. Although Europe is largely Christian, the occupation of south Eastern Europe by the Ottomans resulted in a large Muslim population in Turkey and some Balkan states, even though religion was prohibited in the former Yugoslavia during the communist era. Immigration from those countries has made Islam one of the largest of the European religions. Inter-ethnic conflicts have occurred in a number of areas of south-east Europe, mainly the former Yugoslavia.

Population

The locally dominant population in many countries in Europe is generally old and there is widespread use of contraception. The population is slowly increasing with the influx of immigrants and their descendents. Colonialism by Europeans in Africa and Asia in particular has resulted in immigration from those countries and, more recently the dissolution of the Soviet Empire, the Yugoslavian conflicts and the formation and expansion of the European Community has resulted in increased migrations from Eastern Europe, the Balkans and parts of the former USSR.

Religions

Christianity is the main religion overall, but Islam, Hinduism and Judaism are also seen in most countries (Fig 3-11).Catholicism and Orthodoxy are found especially in southern Europe (Fig 3-12).

Languages

There is no common single language in Europe, but English is widely spoken, particularly in northern countries and understood in many, especially by younger people.

Culture

Europe has a very diverse, largely westernised culture and lifestyle and is evolving into the 'United States of Europe', with continuing efforts being made to eliminate barriers to harmonisation. Despite such developments, and most European countries being multicultural, national traits, languages and traditions continue to be preserved and treasured. Most Europeans, while

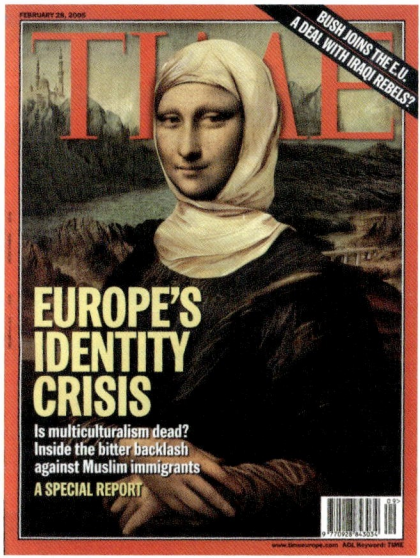

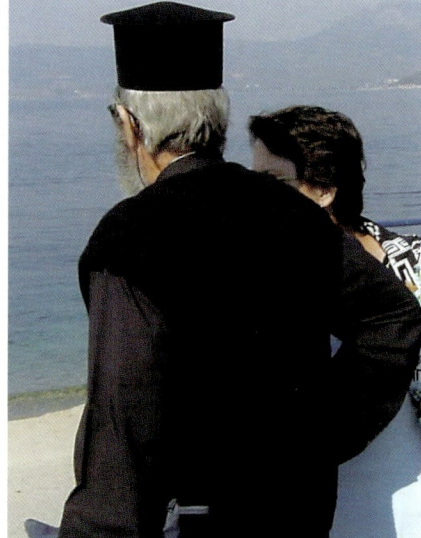

Fig 3-11 Multiculturalism in Europe.　　**Fig 3-12** Greek orthodox priest.

patriotic towards their home country, may increasingly wish to be viewed as becoming more progressive and European.

Overall, family life and culture tends to have at least as much, if not more of an influence on European societies than religious beliefs. Lifestyles are as variable as the peoples and cultures of Europe, but may be considered as southern or northern lifestyles.

As in most other parts of the world, society, culture and lifestyles are changing. A feature of this change is increasing homogeneity; however, national characteristics are anticipated to remain apparent for the foreseeable future. For example, English is increasingly spoken and used in communications, notably in electronic media, including the 'web', but national languages will persist and remain important in many parts of Europe.

Southern Europe
Southern Europeans tend to be very polite and friendly, are typically respectful and often religious. Attitude towards time may be flexible, and work/life balance may favour quality of life. Southern Europeans tend to adopt the so-called Mediterranean lifestyle, characterised by a relatively relaxed approach to everyday affairs. Lunchtime and early afternoon 'siestas' are not uncom-

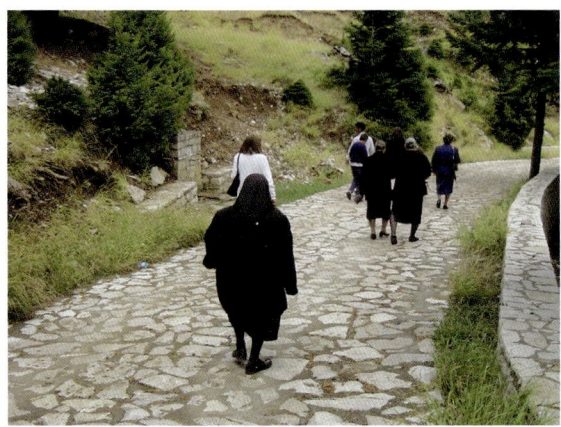

Fig 3-13 Typical black clothing of widows in southern Europe.

mon amongst peoples of Latin descent, and are not always the best times to arrange appointments. Involvement with people and completion of interpersonal encounters is more valued than 'being on time'.

An extended family is common, often including widowed parents (Fig 3-13). Families tend to be patriarchal; the father is the leader, provider, and spokesman; the wife is the carer. There is a strong tradition of mutual support and respect for elders. In family life, elders are respected and children tend to be 'seen but not heard'. Children are sacred but expected to be obedient, and polite to, and respectful of, their elders who, in turn, often help raise the children. Once older people lose their independence, they are typically housed with, and cared for by, their oldest child. Institutionalisation of older people and those with disability is not encouraged.

If hospitalised, they tend to be cared for by family members who take turns at the bedside. Failure to do so may be interpreted as lack of caring. Touching between members of the same sexes is common between southern Europeans and should not be taken to imply anything more than friendship.

Northern Europe
Northern European people are typically polite and distant, and life is often paced according to clock time, which is valued over personal and subjective time. Lifestyles are underpinned by industry and commerce in and around the cities and by agriculture and related service industries in more rural locations.

Families are largely nuclear, with both partners being providers and deci-sion-makers. Respect for parents, elders and authority is less strong than in some other cultures. There is not a strong tradition of mutual support for older people, who are typically housed alone. Institutionalisation of older people and those with disability is not uncommon. If hospitalised, the fam-ily make limited visits but may take turns at the bedside in the event of seri-ous disease.

Northern Europeans may not hide personal feelings and are not reluctant to question decisions, including those of HCPs. Touching between members of the same sexes is less common in northern than southern Europeans, and people of northern European ancestry have a reputation for being somewhat 'cold'.

Dietary and Other Habits and Restrictions
The dietary and other habits and restrictions of Europeans, while still tend-ing to reflect national customs and cuisines, are now very mixed. Overall the diet of Europeans, despite health promotion campaigns, may be found to be conducive to conditions including cardiovascular disease, diabetes and obe-sity, with many diets being cariogenic. Smoking remains prevalent in many European countries, in particular in lower socioeconomic groups and young adults across the social spectrum, notably in the South and East. Health and healthcare provision is, however, a major concession of Europeans of all ages.

Health and Healing Traditions
European countries have most of the health issues of any developed nations. Viruses, bacteria or parasites, which are found throughout Europe, can con-taminate food or water and cause gastroenteritis, hepatitis or other conditions. In Eastern and some Southern areas, viral hepatitis is endemic, and in a few areas tick-borne encephalitis is also endemic in Russia, Czech Republic, Latvia, Lithuania, Estonia, Hungary, Poland, Slovenia, Austria, Germany, Fin-land, Sweden, Switzerland, Denmark (only on the island of Bornholm), and a few cases have also been reported from Italy, Norway, and France. Variant Creutzfeldt-Jakob cases have been reported primarily from the United King-dom, although a small number of cases have been reported from other coun-tries. Large outbreaks of trichinosis have occurred, and in France have been linked to horsemeat. Leishmaniasis (cutaneous and visceral) is found in coun-tries bordering the Mediterranean, with the highest number of cases from Spain, where it is an important opportunistic infection in HIV-infected per-sons. There are serious problems in some areas related to the acquisition, sup-ply and use of drugs of dependence, and their social and health consequences,

with blood-borne infections such as HIV and hepatitis viruses, crime and violence. Tobacco, alcohol, crack and cocaine use are common in many areas. Sexually transmitted infections are on the increase.

Anglo-American values largely pertain (especially in northern Europe) and are summarised by beliefs in individualism, informed consent, science and technology, orientation towards clock time and separation of health from spiritual health significantly affect healthcare. Medicolegal problems and litigation are increasingly commonplace.

Oral Healthcare Issues

Dental care is well accepted throughout Europe. Attitudes and access to dental care may, however, be found to be very variable, with many Europeans, especially from the South and East, either not seeking routine dental care, or being unable to access or afford even basic oral healthcare provision. It is suggested that interest in oral health and, in particular, dental attractiveness is increasing, as evidenced by a steady growth in the range and sale of oral hygiene and related products. As in many parts of the world, there are new emerging dental needs and demands amongst, for example, the elderly who are living longer and retaining more teeth throughout life.

Filipinos

The people of the Philippines are collectively known as Filipinos, a term that originally referred to the Spanish population of the Philippines, but came to be used to refer to the general population of the Southeast Asian country.

History

The Philippines comprises 7,107 islands called the Philippine Archipelago, approximately 700 of which are inhabited. It is the most westernized country in the region, as the Philippines were a Spanish colony for about 350 years and an American colony for 50 years. Filipinos have migrated worldwide, especially to North America, Europe and the Middle East.

Population

The Philippines has one of the most ethnically diverse cultures in the region. Filipinos are predominantly of Malay descent admixed with Chinese, Spanish and American. The Filipino culture is primarily based on the cultures of native groups. Most of the Philippine population (95.5%) descended from Austronesian-speaking immigrants – mainly Tagalog (24%), Cebuanos (24%) and Ilokanos (11%), with the Hiligaynons (Ilonggos), Bikolanos, Waray-Warays,

Kapampangans, Pangasinenses, Kinaray-as, Maranaos, Maguindanaos, and Tausugs. The most significant non-native minorities are ethnic Chinese (1.5%), and expatriate communities of Spaniards, Italians, Poles, other Europeans, Mexicans and Latin Americans, North Americans, Japanese, Koreans, Indians and Pakistanis (Punjabi and Sindhi), Arabs and Vietnamese.

Religions
Most are Christians (95%) (85% Roman Catholics and 10% Protestant churches including Baptists, Evangelicals, Mormons, the Philippine Independent Church and the Iglesia ni Cristo). Minorities are Muslim, Buddhist, Hindus, or Sikhs.

Languages
Pilipino is the national language, but is natively spoken by only one quarter of the population. The Austronesian-speaking immigrants speak their own native dialect. Most Filipinos are literate and fluent in English which is one of the official languages.

Culture
The literacy rate is 96%, one of highest in Asia. Filipinos tend to be warm, friendly, trusting people with a preference to live in large extended families with close family ties. Children tend to be much protected and elders respected.

Greetings
Touch and eye contact tend to be avoided. 'Pagmamano' or placing the right hand of the elder on your forehead is practised as a sign of respect when greeting elders.

Being mostly Christian, Filipinos tend to have a personal name or two followed by a shared family name. Women take their husband's family name on marriage and children take their father's family name.

Dietary and Other Habits and Restrictions
Rice is the Filipinos' staple food, served with all meals. Maize may, however be served as an alternative to rice. Meat, vegetables and, in particular, fish, accompany the rice or maize. Many Filipinos may be lactose intolerant and may avoid wheat products.

Health and Healing Traditions
Eating well is considered to promote health. In general, Filipinos accept

what life brings, tending to believe that all is destined by God. Many Filipinos may be conservative in their expectations of treatment. Modesty and privacy is important to, in particular, Filipino women.

Oral Healthcare Issues
Acceptance of dental care is generally high, with good oral health being viewed as a positive attribute. Elders from villages and barrios chew ' ikmo, bunga at apog' (a white powder and a nut shaped fruit wrapped in a green leaf) and ' nganga' (betel) causing heavy tooth staining. Others traditionally use a sharpened match stick or 'walis tingting' (stick from coconut leaves) as a toothpick, guava branch for cleaning teeth and salt as toothpaste.

In barrios and villages where dentist are not available, people still practice the traditional brushing with salt for toothpaste. Although branded toothpastes are available they are still hardly affordable. In the cities where people are more educated and have more money to spend, they visit the dentist for basic dental treatments.

Japanese
History
In 1603, a military dictatorship ushered in a long period of isolation from foreign influence until 1854, when Japan opened its ports and began to intensively modernize and industrialize becoming a regional power that eventually occupied Korea, Formosa (Taiwan), Manchuria, and China. Between 1877 and 1928, Japanese migrated in large numbers worldwide, especially to the Americas (USA, Canada and Brazil in particular), Europe and the Middle East. In World War II, Japan occupied much of East and Southeast Asia. Japan recovered after its defeat by USA/UK to become an economic power and a staunch ally of the USA, establishing itself as a world economic power. Japan is increasingly recognized as a global strategic power, with Japanese nationals being widely distributed internationally in almost all walks of life, and most strata of society. The roots of Japanese civilization are strong and link the vast majority of Japanese to Japan – 'the land of the rising sun'.

Population
The population of Japan is ethnically homogeneous, with minute populations of North and South Koreans, Okinawan, Chinese, Taiwanese, Filipinos, and Brazilians (mostly of Japanese descent), and the indigenous Ainu in Hokkaido. Japanese have emigrated especially to the Americas (Brazil and USA in particular) and UK.

Religions
Shintoism (54%) or Buddhism (40%). A minority are Christian or have other religions like Shamanism. However, most Japanese people are syncretic, celebrating Shinto rituals, perhaps holding a wedding at a Christian church and a funeral at a Buddhist temple and their concern with religion is usually related to mythology, traditions, and neighbourhood activities. Thus, it is typical for one person or family to believe in several Shinto gods and at the same time belong to a Buddhist sect, and many Japanese homes contain a Buddhist altar (butsudan).

Languages
Japanese, but many Japanese have a good command of English, often a second language for the younger people.

Culture
The Japanese way of life is linked more to tradition and national values than to any religion. The Japanese are widely regarded as very polite and respectful. In communication however, some may exercise self-restraint, avoid eye contact, disagreement and appearing to be unhelpful. Great store may be placed in trust, let alone reassurance of strict confidentiality, notably in respect of personal matters.

Communication is strongly influenced by three main cultural traits, viz;
- Enryo: self-restraint in interacting with others
- Gaman; self-control
- Haji; shame, which must be avoided at all cost.

Japanese tend to be very polite and dislike outward disagreements. This can lead to responses that they believe others want. In addition to Japanese, increasing numbers of Japanese are fluent in English, but head nodding and smiles do not always mean either comprehension or agreement.

Japanese have strong family values with great respect of elders. Children are typically included in family activities and are encouraged to be ambitious in all spheres of their endeavours.

Greetings
Greeting normally consists of a bow, handshake, and use of surname. Japanese may avoid eye contact, and be reserved, and wish to avoid disagreement. Even when an appropriate relationship is established, Japanese may be perceived to be guarded and somewhat formal in their interactions; for exam-

ple, greeting individuals with a bow, handshake and use of title and surname as appropriate.

Dietary and Other Habits and Restrictions
Despite substantial integration internationally, most Japanese maintain a traditional diet of rice supplemented by a wide variety of other foods, in particular, fish and other seafood, pork and poultry. Many Japanese are lactose and alcohol intolerant, relatively few are vegetarian and most will view a balanced diet as important to maintaining good health.

Health and Healing Traditions
Japanese tend to regard time as important and to be fastidious, in particular, in relation to personal hygiene and, while respectful of people in authority, including healthcare professionals, have high expectations of attention to detail and the exercise of care in matters such as professional advice, business transactions and, in healthcare, diagnosis and the provision of treatment best suited to the individual's needs and circumstances. Japanese tend to be punctual for appointments.

The treatment of some chronic conditions may be supplemented by changes to the diet and possibly the adoption of some traditional remedies. Particular attention should be paid to consent, given that most Japanese welcome the opportunity to better understand their conditions and aliments, together with acceptance ('ownership') of the treatment to be provided. In accepting treatment, most Japanese are stoic and reluctant to be troublesome.

Oral Healthcare Issues
Acceptance of dental care is generally high amongst Japanese; however, many Japanese, in particular older Japanese, may not seek routine dental care. Whilst it is impossible to generalise, the people are often conscious of the need for punctuality.

With increasing 'westernisation', Japanese interest in dental attractiveness is increasing.

Kurds

Countries
Kurds are a diverse ethnic group of Indo-Iranian origin inhabiting a mountainous area of Southwest Asia that they call Kurdistan, and that includes parts of Iraq, Turkey, and Iran as well as smaller sections of Syria, Armenia

Table 3-2 **Countries in which Kurds currently mainly live**

Country	Millions of Kurds
Turkey	12
Iraq	4
Iran	4
Syria	1
Germany	0.5
Russia	0.3
Armenia	0.1

and Lebanon (Table 3-2). Often persecuted, Kurds are found in many other parts of the world.

History
Kurds are, together with the people of western and northwestern Iran, widely thought to be descended from the Medes.

Religions
Islam (mostly Sunni). The remaining Kurds are either Christians, Jews or Yezidis (an ancient Kurdish religion).

Languages
Kurdish.

Culture
See Central Asians.

Kurds are quite formal and comment that Anglo-American informality, most importantly the use of first names, is interpreted by all but the most sophisticated Kurds as a sign of weakness, or frivolity. Kurdish women enjoy freedoms not found in more conservative Muslim societies, but their position is still very different from that in many other cultures. Because of their history, Kurds are often wary of laws, regulations and authority, and they may attempt to circumvent regulations.

Dietary and Other Habits and Restrictions
See Central Asians.

Health and Healing Traditions
See Central Asians.

Latin Americans

Central and South America together are often termed Latin, or sometimes Spanish America. The complex culture leads to a special terminology.

Terminology
- 'Creole' – a term with a range of meanings but generally referring to a person with one white and one black parent, born in the Caribbean or Spanish America. Creole languages are those that began as pidgin between a local language and English, French, Spanish, Portuguese, Dutch or Arabic, and then became used as a native language. In Brazil, Crioulo is a black person; a person with one white and one black parent is called Mulato.
- 'Latinos' – just means 'Latin' (which refers to cultures and peoples that can trace their heritage back to the ancient Roman Empire) but it is often (arguably improperly) used to signify those of Spanish or Portuguese descent.
- 'Mestizo' – a Spanish term for peoples of mixed European and Amerindian racial strain inhabiting the region spanning the Americas. Mestizos officially make up the majority of the populations of Paraguay (95%), Venezuela (67%), Ecuador (65%), Mexico (60%) and Colombia (58%). Figures in other countries are lower, with Peru (37%), Bolivia (30%), Argentina (13%), Brazil (12%), and Uruguay (8%). In Portuguese they are termed 'Mestico'.
- 'Zambo' – a Spanish term for Latin Americans of mixed African and Amerindian racial descent. The feminine form is 'Zamba'.

Countries
Argentine, Belize, Bolivia, Brazil, Chile, Colombia, Costa Rica, Ecuador, El Salvador, French Guiana, Guatemala, Guyana, Honduras, Mexico, Nicaragua, Panama, Panama, Paraguay, Peru, Suriname, Uruguay and Venezuela.

History
Spanish colonisation in North, Central and South America (Latin America), except in Brazil - where the Portuguese came, and Guyana/French Guiana colonised by French, British and Dutch had significant detrimental effects on the indigenous (Amerindian) populations. Slavery involving black

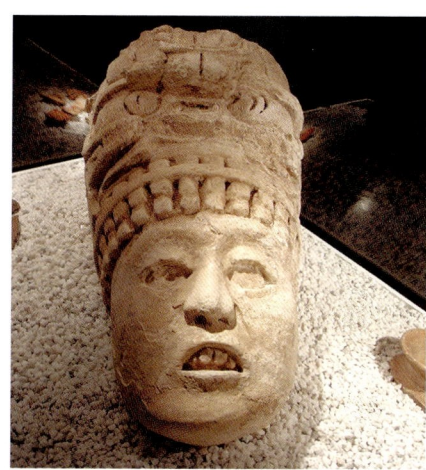

Fig 3-14 Indigenous South American art.

Africans, from West Africa mainly, means that there is a large African American influence, especially in tropical South America. However, the 'Southern Cone' ('Cono Sur': Argentina, Uruguay, Chile, south Brazil), or temperate South America, has historically been largely a European type of culture, based on Spanish, Portuguese, Italian and others, while also admitting many immigrants around the time of the second World War, especially from Poland and Germany.

Population

Indigenous peoples make up the majority of the population in Bolivia, Guatemala and Peru, and are a significant element in most other former Spanish colonies. These Amerindian groups include Awá, Aztecs, Banawa, Caiapos, Enxet, Ge, Incas, Juris, Mapuche, Mayas, Xucuru and Zaparos (Fig 3-14). Exceptions to this include Uruguay and Argentina where, for example, only 10% of the population is Indian.

Spanish descendants predominate in most Latin American countries, except in Brazil, where Portuguese influences predominate. Immigrants from elsewhere have also had significant effects. In the 'Southern Cone' the population and the culture is the most Europeanised of all the Americas.

Africans first arrived with the English, Spanish and Portuguese as slaves. The north of South America has, as a consequence, a population strongly influenced by black African immigration, but the south has been strongly influenced by Spanish, Italians, German and other European immigration. Out-

161

side of the 'Southern Cone', a large percentage of the people are of mixed origins, the result of racial intermingling among European settlers, African slaves and American natives. There are also sizeable communities from other countries, such as Japanese in Brazil. This mixture of backgrounds ('Mestizaje') has profoundly influenced religion, music and politics, and given rise to a vague identity of those belonging to these mixed cultures. This imprecise cultural heritage is called Latinos in American English.

Religions
Christianity (mainly Roman Catholicism) is the primary religion throughout Latin America, but other Christian religions increasing are Protestant, Pentecostal and Evangelical. Buddhism, Judaism, Hinduism and Bahá'í are minority religions, and various Afro-Latin American traditions, such as Santería and Macumba, persist. French Guiana has a large number of Protestants. Guyana and Suriname have three major religions: Christianity, Hinduism and Islam.

Languages
Languages are mainly Spanish (in the nine most populated countries), Portuguese (in Brazil), French (in French Guiana and in some Caribbean countries), English (in Guyana and some Central American and Caribbean countries), Hindi (in Guyana and Suriname), and Dutch and Indonesian (in Suriname). Native languages are also spoken in many Latin American nations, mainly Mexico, Peru and Bolivia. At least three of the Amerindian languages (Guarani in Paraguay, Aymara and Quechua in Peru, Bolivia and Ecuador) are recognised as national languages.

Many nations have their own African-influenced Creole versions of Spanish or other European languages, especially in Central America, Venezuela, Guyana, and French Guiana.

Culture
Latin American peoples are typically very polite, friendly, gracious and hospitable. Latin Americans tend to be respectful and often religious. Attitude towards time may be flexible, and work/life balance may favour quality of life. Involvement with people and completion of interpersonal encounters is more valued than 'being on time'.

An extended family is common, often including widowed parents. Families tend to be patriarchal; the father is the leader, provider, and spokesman; the wife is the carer. There is a strong tradition of mutual support and respect for elders. In family life, elders are respected and children tend to be 'seen but not heard'. Children are sacred, but expected to be obedient, and polite to, and respectful of, their elders who, in turn, often help raise the children. Once older people lose their independence, they are typically housed with, and cared for by, their oldest child. Institutionalisation of older people and those with disability is not encouraged. If hospitalised, they tend to be cared for by family members who take turns at the bedside. Failure to do so may be interpreted as lack of caring.

Dietary and Other Habits and Restrictions
Increasingly, the diet may be formed to be a mixture of traditional and western foods and dishes.

Health and Healing Traditions
The population is rapidly increasing in most countries, but resources are scarce and the per capita income is very low. The population is largely young, and life expectation is predictably lower than in the westernised societies. Outside of the 'Southern Cone', Latin America has a significant proportion of countries that are developing nations. These are mainly in tropical South America. Health risks are generally greater in these areas.

Malnutrition is common in many areas. Yellow fever is present mainly in Panama. Malaria is endemic, as are other parasitic infections. Gnathostomiasis (roundworms) is found in Mexico. Dengue, filariasis, leishmaniasis, onchocerciasis, and American trypanosomiasis (Chagas disease) are diseases carried by insects in the region. Paracoccidioidomycosis is endemic in Brazil and Venezuela. Myiasis (botfly) is endemic in Central America. Viruses, bacteria or parasites found throughout this region can contaminate food or water and cause diarrhoea and vomiting (*E. coli*, salmonella, cholera, and parasites), fever (typhoid fever and toxoplasmosis), or liver damage (hepatitis). Viral hepatitis is endemic. Epidemics of viral encephalitis and dengue fever occur in some countries in this area. Bartonellosis, or Oroya fever (a sandfly-borne disease) occurs in arid river valleys on the western slopes of the Andes. Louse-borne typhus, a rickettsial infection, is often found in mountain areas of Colombia and Peru. Schistosomiasis, a parasitic infection, is found in Brazil, Suriname and north-central Venezuela. Rodent-borne hantavirus pulmonary syndrome has been identified in the north-central and southwestern regions of Argentina and in Chile. There are serious problems in some areas (particularly Colombia and large cities elsewhere) related to the acquisition, supply and use of drugs of dependence, and their social and health consequences, with blood-borne infections such as HIV and hepatitis viruses, TB, crime and violence (Fig 3-15).

163

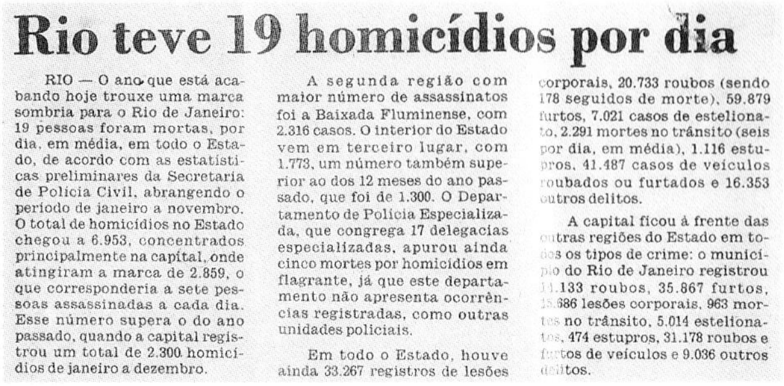

Rio teve 19 homicídios por dia

RIO — O ano-que está acabando hoje trouxe uma marca sombria para o Rio de Janeiro: 19 pessoas foram mortas, por dia, em média, em todo o Estado, de acordo com as estatísticas preliminares da Secretaria de Polícia Civil, abrangendo o período de janeiro a novembro. O total de homicídios no Estado chegou a 6.953, concentrados principalmente na capital, onde atingiram a marca de 2.859, o que corresponderia a sete pessoas assassinadas a cada dia. Esse número supera o do ano passado, quando a capital registrou um total de 2.300 homicídios de janeiro a dezembro.

A segunda região com maior número de assassinatos foi a Baixada Fluminense, com 2.316 casos. O interior do Estado vem em terceiro lugar, com 1.773, um número também superior ao dos 12 meses do ano passado, que foi de 1.300. O Departamento de Polícia Especializada, que congrega 17 delegacias especializadas, apurou ainda cinco mortes por homicídios em flagrante, já que este departamento não apresenta ocorrências registradas, como outras unidades policiais.

Em todo o Estado, houve ainda 33.267 registros de lesões corporais, 20.733 roubos (sendo 178 seguidos de morte), 59.879 furtos, 7.021 casos de estelionato, 2.291 mortes no trânsito (seis por dia, em média), 1.116 estupros, 41.487 casos de veículos roubados ou furtados e 16.353 outros delitos.

A capital ficou à frente das outras regiões do Estado em todos os tipos de crime: o município do Rio de Janeiro registrou 9.133 roubos, 35.867 furtos, 386 lesões corporais, 963 mortes no trânsito, 5.014 estelionatos, 474 estupros, 31.178 roubos e furtos de veículos e 9.036 outros delitos.

Fig 3–15 19 murders each day in Rio de Janeiro .

Outside of the 'Southern Cone', Latin Americans often have a different view of the importance of time and punctuality to Anglo-Americans. If the importance of healthcare appointments is stressed this is not generally a problem. Being on time is often less valued than interpersonal encounters. Early afternoon 'siestas' are not uncommon. Appointments are best avoided at this time.

Latin Americans are often private and modest people who could be most unhappy if their condition were to be discussed with family or friends without their express consent. Same-gender HCPs may be preferred. It is not uncommon that nurses are expected to be female. Interpreters may not be trusted if the patient does not believe they will convey the intended messages, and then family may be preferred over friends to maintain confidentiality. They may have some difficulty understanding why consent should be written and signed.

Adoption of preventive care may be limited. Some systems of healing are built upon indigenous beliefs and traditions, and patients may hold very different understandings of health and disease. The patient may expect the HCP to have all the answers and make all the decisions. As a result, the patient takes a passive role, answering but not asking questions, and waiting for the HCP to impart their diagnosis and recommendations. Most of the time medical and dental advice is accepted without question. Patients may regard as sensitive issues, matters that are sometimes more freely discussed by Western patients. Head-nodding and smiles do not always signify comprehension or agreement; some patients are reluctant to openly disagree with HCPs.

Self-diagnosis and self-treatment are not uncommon. Home remedies may be used extensively, possibly together with prescribed treatments. Patients may have a fear of surgery. If the western treatment fails to bring immediate relief of the symptoms, the patient may seek the care of a traditional

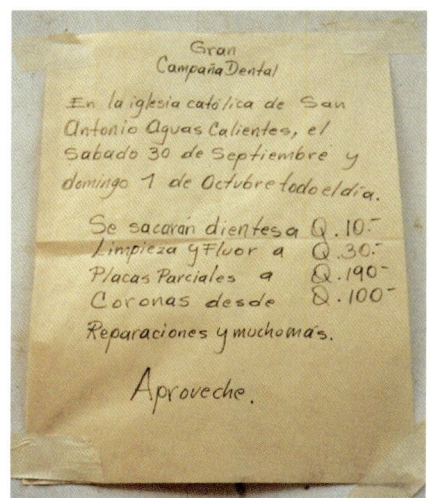

Fig 3-16 Advertisement in Guatemala for dental care.

physician or healer. The same thing may happen if a western diagnosis is rejected because it bears a negative prognosis (including diagnosis of a long-term illness or of an illness that cannot be fully cured) or includes surgery. The traditional treatment may either replace the Western treatment or be used along with it. Many patients do not disclose the use of traditional care and medications to their Western HCPs because the two medical domains - Western and traditional medicine - are seen as entirely separate. Some patients may fear that the Western HCP (an authority figure) will disapprove, or believe that disclosure of the traditional care would violate the relationship of trust.

Many (particularly in the 'Southern Cone'), however, have Anglo-American values summarised by beliefs in individualism, informed consent, science and technology, orientation towards clock time and separation of health from spiritual beliefs.

Oral Healthcare Issues

Outside of the 'Southern Cone', in terms of oral healthcare patients may hold different understandings of health and disease from Westerners. Some patients may, due to cultural or historical experiences, expect tooth conservation but others may expect extraction. High prices or lack of access to treatment, may lead to neglect of dental care where this is not seen as a priority. Dental care is generally accepted, but may only be sought when in pain or discomfort (Fig 3-16).

North Americans

Countries
United States and Canada.

History
British, French and Spanish influences are seen in North America, but slavery involving black Africans, mainly from West Africa, means that there is a large African American influence in USA, especially in the southern states. Immigrants from elsewhere, especially Europe and Asia, have also had significant effects.

Population
This is heterogeneous and consists of:
- Caucasians – those white peoples having origins in any of the original races of Europe, the Middle East, or North Africa
- Hispanics – anybody from or with forebears from Spain or Spanish-speaking Latin America
- People of African descent – those having origins in any of the Black racial groups of Africa
- Asian – frequently of Chinese, Filipino, Indian, Korean or Japanese origin
- Hawaiian/other Pacific Islanders – those having origins in any of the original peoples of Hawaii, Guam, Samoa, or other Pacific Islands
- Native American – those having origins in any of the original peoples of North, Central and South America, and who maintain tribal affiliation or community attachment - American Indians and Alaskan natives

Religions
The primary religion throughout Northern America is Christianity (Roman Catholics, Protestants, Pentecostals, Evangelicals, Mormons, Adventists). Buddhism, Judaism, Hinduism and Bahá'í are indigenous, together with various Afro-Latin American traditions and Islam.

Languages
English, Spanish and French.

Culture
Lifestyles in Northern America are underpinned by industry and commerce in and around the cities and by agriculture and related service industries in rural locations. Despite diversity in culture, language, etiquette and social

interactions, there are many cultural commonalities amongst the people of North America.

North American people of northern European ancestry are typically consumer-orientated. Life is often paced according to clock time. People of Northern European ancestry have a reputation for being somewhat 'colder' than those of other extractions (see Latin Americans, Africans). North American families are largely nuclear. Both partners tend to be providers and decision-makers. Respect for parents, elders and authority is less strong than in some cultures. There is not a strong tradition of mutual support for older people, who are often housed alone. Institutionalisation of older people and those with disability is not uncommon. If hospitalised, the family make limited visits, but may take turns at the bedside.

North Americans may not reveal personal feelings, but are not reluctant to question decisions, including those of HCPs. Medicolegal problems and litigation are commonplace.

As in most other parts of the world, society, culture and lifestyles are changing in North America. A feature of this change is increasing homogeneity; however, national characteristics are anticipated to remain apparent for the foreseeable future. For example, English is often used in communications, notably in electronic media, including the 'web', but Spanish is becoming increasingly important in the USA as it is in Mexico. French will persist in Canada.

Dietary and Other Habits and Restrictions
The dietary and other habits and restrictions of North Americans are now very mixed. Overall the diet of North Americans, despite health promotion campaigns, may be found to be conducive to conditions including cardiovascular disease, diabetes and obesity, with many diets being cariogenic. Smoking remains prevalent in most North American countries, in particular in lower socioeconomic groups and young adults across the social spectrum. Alcohol consumption is widespread.

Health and Healing Traditions
Canada and the USA have most of the health issues of any developed nations. Viruses, bacteria or parasites, which are found throughout the region can contaminate food or water and may cause diarrhoea and vomiting (*E. coli*, salmonella, cholera, and parasites), fever (typhoid fever and toxoplasmosis)

or liver damage (hepatitis). Certain diseases occasionally occur, such as plague, rabies in wildlife - including bats, raccoons, foxes, and other wild animals - Rocky Mountain spotted fever, tularemia and arthropod-borne encephalitis. Coccidioidomycosis is endemic in southwestern United States. Histoplasmosis is highly endemic, especially in the Mississippi, Ohio and the St. Lawrence River valleys.

Rodent-borne Hantavirus pulmonary syndrome has been identified, predominantly in the western states of the United States. Lyme disease is endemic in the northeastern United States, Mid-Atlantic, and the upper Midwest and the southwestern provinces of Canada. Recently, cases of West Nile virus have occurred throughout North America. During recent years, the incidence of certain foodborne diseases, e.g. *E. coli* O157:H7 and salmonellosis, has increased in some regions. Although the risk of hepatitis A infection is low in the United States and Canada, outbreaks have occurred in some areas. Isolated cases of bovine spongiform encephalopathy (BSE/mad cow disease) have been reported in Canada and the United States.

Anglo-American values are summarised by individualism, expectation of informed consent, science and technology, orientation towards clock time and separation of health from spiritual beliefs. Whilst it is impossible to generalise, the people are often conscious of the need for punctuality. Health and healthcare provision is, however, a major concern of North Americans of all ages.

There are serious problems in some areas related to the acquisition, supply and use of drugs of dependence, and their social and health consequences, with blood-borne infections such as HIV and hepatitis viruses, crime and violence. Alcohol, crack, cocaine and heroin use are common in many areas. Sexually transmitted infections are on the increase.

Oral Healthcare Issues

Dental care is well accepted throughout North America. Attitudes and access to dental care may, however, be found to be very variable, with many North Americans either not seeking routine dental care, or being unable to access or afford even basic oral healthcare provision. It is suggested that interest in oral health and, in particular, dental attractiveness is increasing, as evidenced by a steady growth in the range and sale of oral hygiene and related products.

As in many parts of the world, there are new emerging dental needs and demands amongst, for example, the elderly who are living longer and retaining more teeth throughout life.

168

Roma/Gypsies

Roma is the preferred term when referring to people commonly, but incorrectly, known as Gypsies.

'New Age Travellers' are not Roma, but usually British or Irish itinerants.

Countries
Most Roma are in Romania, Bosnia, Bulgaria, Kosovo (a province of Serbia) and Slovakia.

History
The Roma are believed to have originated in India about AD 1000, and to have passed through what is now Afghanistan, Persia, Armenia and Turkey to the Balkans, *en route* to the UK, Scandinavia, USA and Latin America.

Religions
There is no separate Romani religion, rather the Roma traditionally adopt the dominant religion of the country in which they live, and most therefore are Christian. However, in Macedonia and Kosovo they have been particularly active in Islamic mystical brotherhoods (Sufism).

Languages
Romani – derived primarily from Sanskrit. English (sometimes Greek, Russian, Serbian or Spanish) may be spoken. Roma not infrequently cannot read or write.

Culture
Roma are generally a nomadic people with an alternative lifestyle and reluctance to conform. They are typically mistrustful of non-Roma and do not like touch, especially to the head. They often wear an amulet around the neck, which should not be removed without permission.

Roma are very respectful to their elders, family involvement is strong and there is often a spokesperson, typically a parent. Roma men make the decisions but the women make money and communicate medical knowledge.

Romany social behaviour is strictly regulated by purity laws ('marime'), and they take virginity very seriously. This regulation affects many aspects of life, and is applied to actions, people and things. The genital organs, because they produce impure emissions, and the lower body are considered impure,

169

and clothes for the lower body, and all clothes of menstruating women must be washed separately. Items used for eating are also washed in a different place. Childbirth is considered impure, and must occur outside the dwelling place; the mother is considered impure during 40 days. Death is seen as impure as well and affects the whole family of the dead, who remain impure for a period of time.

Dietary and Other Habits and Restrictions

Roma on Fridays often eat fish, or at least no animal products. A large percentage of Roma smoke and have high calorific diets, putting them at increased risk of hypertension, occlusive vascular disease, strokes, myocardial infarctions and diabetes.

Health and Healing Traditions

Attitudes towards disease prevention and screening are often poor. Orientation towards time is typically limited. Involvement with people and completion of interpersonal encounters is more valued than 'being on time'. Understanding of disease pathogenesis is variable and there may be strong beliefs that the Devil causes many illnesses. Crowded living conditions lead to an increased incidence of gastrointestinal and respiratory infections. Social isolation leads to an increase in consanguineous marriages, and thus an increased risk for birth defects.

In the healthcare setting, only the elder males of some groups are likely to communicate with HCPs. Women are not permitted to interrupt men or to be alone with a man who is not their husband or relative. They therefore prefer same-gender HCPs. Roma are also often suspicious of HCPs, respecting older, not young practitioners.

Roma often become anxious if ill, especially about cancer and death, and fearful of general anesthesia and surgery. When a clan member must enter a hospital, family members are expected to remain with that person day and night to watch over, protect and perform caring and curing rituals. Women are the main carers. They may ignore medical advice.

Washing hands after touching the lower body before touching the upper body is required. Separate soap and towels are used on the upper and lower parts of the body and they must not be allowed to mix.

Roma share common folk beliefs that include the sanctity of a deceased person's body. There are therefore restrictions on donations of blood or organs.

The soul retains a physical shape and all body parts must be left intact. They tend to associate cancer with death.

Roma often stop medication too soon. Older women in the community may be healers (drabarnis).

Oral Healthcare Issues
The negative attitudes of Roma to prevention are not conducive to good oral health. Furthermore, Roma dislike general anaesthesia and surgery; they are especially fearful of any surgical procedure that requires general anaesthesia because of belief that a person under general anaesthesia undergoes a 'little death'. For the family to gather around the person recovering from general anaesthesia is especially important.

South Asians

South Asia is synonymous with the term Indian sub-continent, one of the most densely populated areas of the world, where one quarter of the world population lives.

Countries
South Asia is usually taken to include a number of developing countries such as Bangladesh, Bhutan, India, Maldives, Nepal, Pakistan and Sri Lanka.

History
Much of South Asia was colonised by Britain before the Indian sub-continent was partitioned into India (largely Hindu), East Pakistan (now Bangladesh – largely Muslim), and West Pakistan (now Pakistan – also Muslim). There are continuing tensions between India and Pakistan, and in Sri Lanka between Singalhese and Tamils. South Asians have migrated widely, especially to East Africa, Fiji, the Middle East, the Caribbean, UK and North America.

Population
South Asians are a people of great ethnic and religious diversity, as indicated above.

Religions
Hinduism, Islam, Buddhism, Jainism and Sikhism predominate.

Languages
English is widely spoken and used largely for national, political, legal and

commercial purposes. The other main languages are Urdu, Hindi, Punjabi, Gujarati, Bengali and Tamil.

Culture
South Asians are typically modest, respectful, friendly, gracious and hospitable. Touching is uncommon. Modesty, humility and shyness are admired: direct eye contact may be avoided as it can be considered disrespectful, especially towards older people. Silence usually indicates acceptance, approval or tolerance.

South Asians are often religious. Their attitude towards time may be somewhat flexible, and work/life balance may favour quality of life, but appointment keeping is respected.

Families tend to be patriarchal. The father is responsible for matters outside the home, the leader, provider and spokesman; the wife is the carer and responsible for activities within the home. Decisions are often shared. An extended family is common, often including widowed parents. Daughters are expected to move in with the husband's family on marriage. There is a strong tradition of mutual support and respect for elders. In family life, elders are respected and children tend to be 'seen but not heard'. Children are sacred but expected to be obedient, and polite to, and respectful of, their elders who, in turn, often help raise the children. Older people are typically housed with, and cared for by, their oldest child, preferably a married son. Institutionalisation of older people or those with disability is not encouraged.

There is a huge variation in dress, ranging from strict codes to casual Western style. Older generations often wear traditional Indian clothing that is common for others on special occasions.

Non-verbal gestures are part of day-to-day communication.

Dietary and Other Habits and Restrictions
The cuisine revolves around religion, custom and place of origin and is characterised by the use of many, varied spices. The staple food ranges from bread made from wheat flour (chapattis) to rice of different types. Meat consumption is largely determined according to religious belief; Hindus and Sikhs eat no beef, Muslims eat no pork, and Jains and Buddhists eat no meat.

Betel use is common throughout South Asia. Indian men may smoke or chew tobacco, but alcohol, if taken at all, is generally consumed in moderation. Indian women and most Sikhs do not smoke tobacco or drink alcohol.

Health and Healing Traditions

South Asian countries are mainly developing nations. The populations are rapidly increasing, but resources are scarce and malnutrition is common. Inter-ethnic conflicts are on-going in some areas. The population is largely young. Life expectation is predictably lower than in westernised societies. Malaria is endemic, as are other parasitic infections and TB. HIV is rapidly increasing.

Food and waterborne diseases can be caused by viruses, bacteria, or parasites, which are found throughout South Asia. Diarrhoea and vomiting (*E. coli*, salmonella, cholera, and parasites), fever (typhoid fever and toxoplasmosis) or liver damage (hepatitis) are common. Typhoid fever can be contracted through contaminated drinking water or food, or by eating food or drinking beverages that have been handled by a person who is infected. Large outbreaks are most often related to faecal contamination of water supplies or foods sold by street vendors. *Salmonella typhi* strains resistant to multiple antibiotics are found in this region: there have been recent reports of typhoid drug resistance in India and Nepal. Filariasis is common in Bangladesh, India, and Sri Lanka. A sharp rise in the incidence of visceral leishmaniasis has been seen in Bangladesh, India, Nepal and Pakistan, where it is mainly reported from the north (Baltisan). Cutaneous leishmaniasis occurs in Afghanistan, India (Rajasthan) and Pakistan. Dengue fever can occur in Bangladesh, India, Pakistan and Sri Lanka. Japanese encephalitis occurs widely except in mountainous areas. Polio is endemic in India and Afghanistan. Rabies is common in the region. Leptospirosis, a bacterial infection often contracted through recreational water activities in contaminated water, is common in tropical areas of this region.

Peoples of these cultures may view health and disease and healthcare in a strikingly different fashion from Anglo-Americans. Indeed, entire systems of healing are built upon indigenous beliefs and traditions and patients may hold very different understandings of health and disease. Involvement with people and completion of interpersonal encounters is more valued than 'being on time'. The patient may expect the HCP to have all the answers and make all the decisions. As a result, the patient takes a passive role, answering but not asking questions, and waiting for the HCP to impart their diagnosis and recommendations. Most of the time medical and dental advice is accepted without question. Patients may regard as sensitive issues, matters which are sometimes more freely discussed by Westernized patients. Head-nodding and smiles do not always signify comprehension or agreement; some patients are reluctant openly to disagree with HCPs.

If the Western treatment fails to bring immediate relief of the symptoms, the patient may seek the care of a traditional physician or healer. The same thing may happen if a Western diagnosis is rejected because it bears a negative prognosis (including diagnosis of a long-term illness or of an illness that cannot be fully cured) or because surgery is advised. The traditional treatment may either replace the Western treatment or be used along with it. Many patients do not disclose the use of traditional care and medications to their Western HCPs because the two medical domains are seen as separate. Some patients may also fear that the Western HCP will disapprove, or believe that disclosure of the traditional care would violate the relationship of trust. If hospitalised, they tend to be cared for by family who take turns at the bedside. Failure to do so may be interpreted as lack of caring.

Oral Healthcare Issues
Knowledge of dental matters and the importance of oral health may be limited and patients may hold very different understandings of health and disease. While the acceptance of Western healthcare, including dentistry, is widespread, the uptake of dental care may be limited. Given the high incidence of cardiovascular disease and diabetes, in particular amongst elderly people, there may be anxieties about the risks of treatment. It is generally best to ask direct questions about such concerns and the use of traditional medicines, which may mask certain diseases and conditions, or complicate the treatment.

High prices, or lack of access to treatment may lead to neglect of dental care, in particular, where this is not seen as a priority. Some patients may, due to cultural or historical experiences, expect tooth extractions but others may expect conservation.

South East Asians

Countries
The countries of South East Asia include Brunei, Cambodia, East Timor, Indonesia, Laos, Malaysia, Myanmar (Burma), Philippine, Singapore, Thailand (Siam) and Vietnam. The mainland area was formerly termed Indochina. The Association of Southeast Asian Nations (ASEAN), established in 1967 and now including Indonesia, Malaysia, Philippines, Singapore, Thailand, Brunei Darussalam, Vietnam, Laos, Myanmar and Cambodia, aims to accel-

erate the economic growth, social progress and cultural development in the region through joint endeavours in the spirit of equality and partnership to strengthen the foundation for a prosperous and peaceful community of Southeast Asian nations. A further aim is to promote stability through abiding respect for justice and the rule of law, with adherence to the principles of the United Nations Charter.

History
South East Asia has suffered from the effects of colonialization by British, French, Dutch and Japanese, and from several conflicts involving China, Japan and the USA. Many of the countries are resource-poor and tropical.

Population
The peoples are diverse in Southeast Asia and not one country is homogenous.

Religions
Islam, Hinduism, Christianity, Buddhism, and Animism are the predominant religions. In the world's most populous Muslim nation, Indonesia, Hinduism is dominant on islands such as Bali, but Balinese Hinduism is somewhat different from Hinduism practised elsewhere – as Animism and local culture are incorporated. Pockets of Hindu population exist in Singapore, Malaysia etc. Christianity predominates in Timor and the Philippines. In Vietnam, the form of Mahayana Buddhism practiced is heavily influenced by the Animism and tribal religions of the native peoples. Indigenous tribal religious practices are found in Sarawak, East Malaysia and Irian Jaya in eastern Indonesia.

Languages
The languages spoken include, on mainland Southeast Asia: Khmer, Vietnamese, Thai, various Chinese dialects, Burmese and Lao/Isan; on the Malay archipelago, the family of Austronesian languages (the most widely dispersed language family in the world, geographically) includes: Malay, the Indonesian languages, the Philippine languages, and so forth. Within each of these languages, there are many local dialects. There are also many other languages spoken by tribal peoples.

Culture
South East Asians are a people of tremendous ethnic and religious diversity, culture and tradition but with a strong Chinese influence.

Modesty, humility and shyness are admired. Direct eye contact may be avoided as it can be considered disrespectful, especially towards older people, but lowered eyes are acceptable. Pointing is also considered disrespectful. Silence usually indicates acceptance and approval or tolerance. There is a tradition of saving face. The people are typically respectful, friendly, gracious and hospitable. Gentle touching is common, but never of the head. It is acceptable for heterosexual men or women to hold hands with same gender. Personal space may be more than for Anglo-Americans.

South East Asians are often religious. Attitude towards time may be somewhat flexible, and work/life balance may favour quality of life, but appointment keeping is generally respected.

Families tend to be patriarchal. The father is responsible for decisions, matters outside the home, the leader, provider, and spokesman; the wife is the carer and responsible for activities within the home, may work, and often influences the husband's decisions. An extended family is common, often including several generations in the same home. Daughters are expected to move in with the husband's family on marriage. There is a strong tradition of mutual support and respect for elders. In family life, elders are respected and children tend to be 'seen but not heard'. Children are sacred, but expected to be obedient, and respectful of, their elders who, in turn, often help raise the children and prepare meals for the family. Older people are typically housed with and cared for by their oldest child, preferably a married son. Institutionalisation of older people and those with disability is disrespectful. If hospitalised, they tend to be cared for by family who take turns at the bedside. Failure to do so may be interpreted as lack of caring.

Dietary and Other Habits and Restrictions
The people typically use chopsticks and take a rice-based diet, often with soy sauce and ample vegetables. They tend to dislike cold foods. They are often lactose-intolerant. They tend to believe hot/cold properties are inherent in foods and may influence health. Betel use is common.

Health and Healing Traditions
South East Asia has developed westernized societies such as in Singapore, and a significant proportion of the countries are developing nations. The population is rapidly increasing in most countries and is largely young. Inter-ethnic conflicts are on-going in some areas.

Malaria is endemic as are other parasitic infections and TB. HIV is increasing. Diarrhoea can be caused by viruses, bacteria, or parasites, found throughout Southeast Asia and can contaminate food or water. Infections may cause diarrhoea and vomiting (*E. coli*, salmonella, cholera, and parasites), fever (typhoid fever and toxoplasmosis), or liver damage (hepatitis). Dengue, filariasis, Japanese encephalitis, and plague are diseases carried by insects that occur in this region. Avian influenza H5N1 is also present. Polio has resurfaced in Indonesia. Rabies is common. Schistosomiasis is seen in certain areas of Cambodia, Indonesia, Laos, Philippines, and Thailand. Leptospirosis, a bacterial infection often contracted through activities in contaminated water, is common in tropical areas of this region.

South East Asians may view health and disease and healthcare in a strikingly different fashion from Anglo-Americans. Their systems of healing are built upon indigenous beliefs and traditions.

Being on time is often less valued than personal attention. Involvement with people and completion of interpersonal encounters is more valued than 'being on time'. The patient may expect the HCP to have all the answers and make all the decisions. As a result, the patient takes a passive role, answering but not asking questions, and waiting for the HCP to impart their diagnosis and recommendations. Most of the time medical and dental advice is accepted without question. Patients may regard as sensitive issues, matters that are sometimes more freely discussed by westernised patients. Head-nodding and smiles do not always signify comprehension or agreement; some patients are reluctant openly to disagree with HCPs.

Traditional Chinese medicine is often used, alone or along with Western treatment. A Western diagnosis may be rejected because it bears a negative prognosis (including diagnosis of a long-term illness or of an illness that cannot be fully cured) or because surgery is advised. Many patients do not disclose the use of traditional care and medications to their western HCPs because the two medical domains are seen as separate. Some patients may fear that the Western HCP will disapprove, or believe that disclosure of the traditional care would violate the relationship of trust.

Oral Healthcare Issues
While the acceptance of western healthcare, including dentistry, is increasingly widespread, the uptake of, in particular, dental care may be limited and advanced disease may present (Fig 3–17). Given the high incidence of cardiovascular disease and diabetes, in particular amongst elderly people, there may be anxieties about the risks of treatment. It is generally best to ask direct

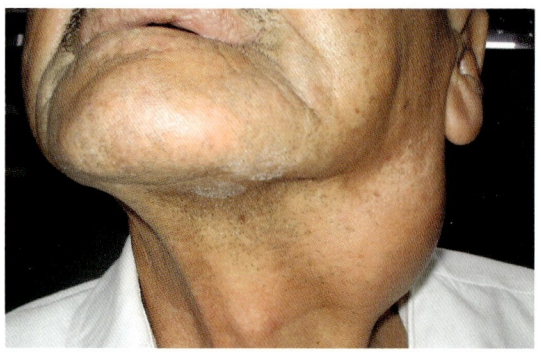

Fig 3-17 Advanced metastatic oral cancer.

questions about such concerns and the use of traditional medicines, which may mask certain diseases and conditions or complicate treatment.

Knowledge of dental matters and the importance of oral health may be limited, and patients may hold very different understandings of health and disease. Some patients may, due to cultural or historical experiences, expect extraction, but others may expect tooth conservation. High prices or lack of access to treatment may lead to neglect of dental care, in particular, where this is not seen as a priority.

Cultures and Countries

Countries of the world, with some notable exceptions, are increasingly multicultural, with growing ethnic minority groups practising their religions and beliefs to varying extents and degrees within and between different countries. Despite this multiculturalisation, national identities have largely been maintained but possibly somewhat modified by changing circumstances and population profiles. As a consequence, country of origin or residence may not be found to be such an important factor in cultural considerations in healthcare as it may have been in times gone by. Notwithstanding such change, knowledge and understanding of religious, political, cultural and social customs and practices in the many different countries of the world can help inform culturally sensitive healthcare. Consideration of such diversity is outwith the scope of this relatively brief text. However, providers of healthcare, including oral healthcare, are encouraged to learn and understand more of the countries their patients originated from or have been influenced by during some period of residency. As in all other aspects of cultural assessment, patients must be treated as individuals, never stereotyped by, for example, nationality. This highlights the need to be effective in communicating with patients and understanding the needs and wishes of the individual if healthcare provision is to be culturally sensitive. Above all else the healthcare profession must never discriminate against a patient for whatever reason.

Websites and Further Reading

http://www.cdc.gov/travel/destinat.htm (Centers for Disease Control and Prevention: guide for travelers)

http://en.wikipedia.org/wiki/Culture#Cultures_of_contemporary_countries_and_regions (Encyclopaedia entry definition of culture in terms of civilizations, values, norms, artifacts, products and activities)

http://www.nativeweb.org (Resources for indigenous cultures around the world, including health)
http://www.omhrc.gov/cultural/completed.htm (The centre for linguistic and cultural competence in healthcare)

Further Reading

Bussey-Jones J, Genao I. Impact of culture on healthcare. J Natl Med Assoc 2003; 95:8,732-735.

Kleinman, A. Patients and Healers in the Context of Culture. Berkeley. University of California Press, 1980.

MacLachlan M. Culture and Health. Chichester: John Wiley and Sons, 1997

Index

Quintessentials for General Dental Practitioners Series

in 50 volumes

Editor-in-Chief: Professor Nairn H F Wilson

General Dentistry, Editor: Nairn Wilson

Implantology in General Dental Practice	available
Culturally Sensitive Oral Healthcare	available
Dental Erosion	available
Managing Orofacial Pain in Practice	Autumn 2006
Dental Bleaching	Autumn 2006
Special Care Dentistry	Autumn 2006
Infection Control for the Dental Team	Spring 2007
Therapeutics and Medical Emergencies in the Everyday Clinical Practice of Dentistry	Spring 2007

Oral Surgery and Oral Medicine, Editor: John G Meechan

Practical Dental Local Anaesthesia	available
Practical Oral Medicine	available
Practical Conscious Sedation	available
Minor Oral Surgery in Dental Practice	available

Imaging, Editor: Keith Horner

Interpreting Dental Radiographs	available
Panoramic Radiology	available
Twenty-first Century Dental Imaging	Autumn 2006

Periodontology, Editor: Iain L C Chapple

Understanding Periodontal Diseases: Assessment and Diagnostic Procedures in Practice	available
Decision-Making for the Periodontal Team	available
Successful Periodontal Therapy – A Non-Surgical Approach	available
Periodontal Management of Children, Adolescents and Young Adults	available
Periodontal Medicine: A Window on the Body	available

Endodontics, Editor: John M Whitworth

Rational Root Canal Treatment in Practice	available
Managing Endodontic Failure in Practice	available
Restoring Endodontically Treated Teeth	Autumn 2006

Prosthodontics, Editor: P Finbarr Allen

Teeth for Life for Older Adults	available
Complete Dentures – from Planning to Problem Solving	available
Removable Partial Dentures	available
Fixed Prosthodontics in Dental Practice	available
Occlusion: A Theoretical and Team Approach	Autumn 2006

Operative Dentistry, Editor: Paul A Brunton

Decision-Making in Operative Dentistry	available
Aesthetic Dentistry	available
Communicating in Dental Practice	available
Indirect Restorations	Summer 2006
Choosing and Using Dental Materials	Autumn 2006

Paediatric Dentistry/Orthodontics, Editor: Marie Therese Hosey

Child Taming: How to Cope with Children in Dental Practice	available
Paediatric Cariology	available
Treatment Planning for the Developing Dentition	available
Managing Dental Trauma in Practice	available

General Dentistry and Practice Management, Editor: Raj Rattan

The Business of Dentistry	available
Risk Management	available
Quality Matters: From Clinical Care to Customer Service	Summer 2006
Practice Management for the Dental Team	Autumn 2006
Dental Practice Design	Autumn 2006
Handling Complaint in Dental Practice	Autumn 2006

Dental Team, Editor: Mabel Slater

Team Players in Dentistry	Autumn 2006

Quintessence Publishing Co. Ltd., London